CW00351181

PELVIC FLOOR
SECRETS

6 weeks to confidence, continence and sexual satisfaction

Jenni Russell

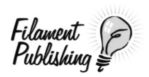

Filament Publishing Ltd
16 Croydon Road
Waddon, Croydon
Surrey CR0 4PA

Telephone: +44 (0)208 688 2598
email: info@filamentpublishing.com
Website: www.filamentpublishing.com

ISBN 978-1-908691-39-2

© Jenni Russell 2012

Illustrations © by Juliet Percival

The right of Jenni Russell to be recognised as the
author of this work has been asserted by her in
accordance with the Copyright and Patents Act 1988.

Printed by the Berforts Information Press
Stevenage and Eastbourne

The book is protected by international copyright
and may not be reproduced in any way without the
prior written consent of the publishers.

Table of Contents

Acknowledgements

THE greatest and biggest thanks go to my Heavenly Father, God. Without His grace, mercy and unfailing love, I would not be able to use the gift and talent He placed in me to be a blessing to others. The gift of exhortation allows me to educate and encourage, empower and excite women (and men) about their future. I am always mindful that all things are possible through Christ who strengthens me.

When I first began this journey towards putting this second book together, I had not yet met my partner, Tony. What a subject for a man to walk into! Thank you for helping me to get this project off the ground. I hope we are able to enjoy the rewards and witness the benefits, not just for ourselves but, from anyone whose life is enhanced by this book. I love you.

I also have to thank my beautiful son Jourdan-Reiss who has been studying for his A2 finals with his head in his books alongside me. I am blessed to have the relationship I have with you. Thanks for helping to come up with the title and for your input into this project. Continue to aim high and success will be your portion.

I have a mother that has supported my craziness forever! She has listened, allowed me to talk about the subject, and sat listening to everything, technical and otherwise, and encouraged me and carried me when I needed it. Thank you Mum, I love you. Dad would have loved this – miss him loads. This book is dedicated to you, Dad. To my brothers and sisters also: Beverley, Colin, Lorna, Brenda and Martin, my sister-in-law Annette and my beautiful niece Sadie-Rose. Everyone has had to listen to this forever and still you listen. Thank you.

Nicky Clarke, an amazing lady and now a dear friend also, found me on the Internet in July 2009 and asked if I would not mind writing an article for her upcoming magazine, *Juno Mum*. It was here that "Va-Va-Voom your Vagina" was born (your title) and this whole topic was revisited. Once you got me going... Thank you so much!

Thanks also to my new surrogate father Vasco Stevenson, who sits on the executive committee of the Association of Prostate Awareness (APA), for his input and information on testicular cancer and prostate issues. May you continue to inform men and keep them well, even through this book. Thanks for your time, energy and patience, and your belief in my delivery of pelvic floor issues for all.

I also want to thank a dear friend, Vince Philgence, for his continued support, input and patience. He has put up with my craziness for many years, helping to boost my business and being an integral part of brand Jenni Russell. I pray your family will be blessed by this success also.

Suzanne Sloan is a friend and colleague. Thank you Suzanne for giving me the sole distribution of such an amazing product, Gyneflex™, and for coming to the UK for my seminar, without asking for a fee, and for reading this project and providing positive feedback. I pray this project elevates the lives of women everywhere and brings our products into every household.

There are many people that I need to thank for their input and patience as I have worked on this project and talked about it over and over. Every time I have discussed it, I have come up with another analogy.

There are too many names to put here, but you do know who you are and I love you all. This book is in loving memory of my best friend from college, Annette Charles, who unfortunately did not win her battle against pancreatic cancer. RIP Annette, my "pin-head posse" friend, I love and will miss you always. Rest in Peace.

Juliet Percival is an amazing woman with an amazing eye and awesome hand that has detailed my book beautifully. Thank you for bringing to life the most precious part of our body in such a sophisticated and delicate way. I thank God for the day I was introduced to you. Thank you for making this book the unique tool that it is.

And last but by no means least to my editor, Mildred Talabi. What a project to sit and read through, edit amazingly and add feedback. Thanks for all your help and ensuring this book will be the success you have the faith for. May our new and continued friendship bless many with more books to come. This book is for every woman and her daughter(s), ensuring confidence and continence and at the appropriate time sexual satisfaction. It is also a must for her husband or partner and her son(s) to ensure their confidence, continence and at the appropriate time sexual satisfaction. Beautifully illustrated and informative – you need never suffer dysfunction because this book gives you all the tools you need. Enjoy and be enlightened.

Foreword

EVERYONE should have a Jenni Russell in his or her life. She is a dynamo of caring and commitment to fitness and strength! She is also un-phased by the things that have most of us reticent Brits curled into a ball of awkwardness. In this beautifully illustrated book, Jenni grabs the bull and gets on with it, with humour and seriousness sandwiched together in a most unlikely combination. And hey presto, suddenly nothing seems embarrassing and everything seems important.

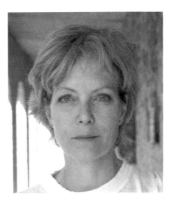

Jenny Seagrove *Actress*

So girls and guys – whatever age you are - join the Pelvic Floor Secrets club. This is the forgotten muscle, and my God, how important it is. I'm not Jenni, so read and enjoy the book for your detail, but just on a purely health and strength basis, with everything else being a bonus (and what a bonus..) take it to heart and do what she says.

Enjoy!

About the author

JENNI Russell is the woman who can make you confident, continent and sexually satisfied in 6 weeks!

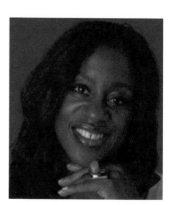

Jenni Russell *Author*

She is CHEK certified: Holistic Nutrition and Lifestyle Coach (Level 1) with over 20 years of personal training experience, and has specialised in pelvic floor health since 1996. Jenni's passion and commitment to pelvic floor health and the desire to give women the access to a service that requires no special creams, medication or surgery, is the reason she opened her own unique pelvic floor clinic in Central London in March 2011. Initially at The Albany Club, the clinic has since grown and moved to her prestigious address 1 Harley Street. Jenni works with women who need her help in a compassionate, un-phased and unique way to produce long lasting and positive results. Client confidence is renewed visibly (especially the shape and function of the butt, thighs and lower abdominals, as well as posture) and intimately with increased continence, support and protection of the organs. Her clients describe her as "life changing".

Jenni's first book, *Can a Vagina Really Buy a Mercedes?* (subtitled, *What can your pelvic floor do for you?*) was featured on ITV's *This Morning* in June 2006 and appeared in the *News of the World Sunday Magazine* as a full page article. She continues to write and speak about pelvic floor health around the country and is a regular contributor to local radio, with BBC London presenter Vanessa Feltz describing her as having an "Obama-like quality."

Jenni is a seasoned athlete, currently holding the title of "Britain's Fittest Woman" after winning the British Ultrafit Championship three times in 1995, 1998 and 2000. In 2000, Jenni took part in the Channel 5 game show *The Desert Forges*, a gruelling challenge of endurance tests set in the scorching Wadi Rum desert in Jordan, and emerged as the overall winner. She has also run both the London and New York Marathon.

With appearances on BBC Two's *Economy Gastronomy* in 2009 and on a cameo role in Channel 4's *Celebrity Wife Swap* in the same year, alongside her client, singer and TV personality Sinitta, Jenni is no stranger to public appearances.

Jenni's mantra is "Be Ready, Be Educated" Pelvic Floor Secrets can give you the confidence to enjoy life without fear of pain or embarrassment. Childbirth does not have to change the way you feel about your sexuality and intimacy. The right education can make motherhood rewarding whether on the trampoline or in the bedroom. It's within your reach.

Preface

True beauty is rarely witnessed!

WHAT do you see when you look at this gorgeous house? Seems like an obvious question, but the true beauty of this image is not what the eye can see, whether inside or out, but something that is rarely thought about.

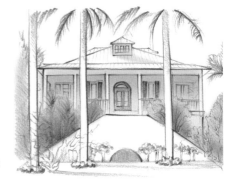

The true beauty is the foundation that this wonderful splendour sits on. It is the foundation that makes the obvious beauty we see possible. The stronger the foundation, the longer the outward beauty can be witnessed. The strongest foundations mean a house such as this can be enjoyed for many generations. The foundation of any building is continually working - it works against the elements and against the load, which is placed upon it on a daily basis. It has the primary role of support and protection, with the rewards of satisfaction, stability and longevity. A strong foundation is the most important part of any building, but for most of us, it is rarely thought about until or unless it begins to let us down!

Just as the foundation of a house must support and protect, so too must the foundation of our torso or trunk. The pelvic floor is the foundation of our torso. It is positioned as a sling right at the bottom of the abdominal cavity, just above the pubic bone in both males and females. This hammock-like set of muscles works constantly against gravity and environmental factors such as sports, excessive lifting, obesity, poor diet choices and so on. The primary role of the pelvic floor is to support and protect the internal organs: supporting them in their anatomical positions within the trunk and protecting against involuntary loss of waste or against organ prolapse. The reproductive organs run straight through the supporting pelvic floor and thus it has a direct relationship and part to play in the strength and function of both the vagina and the penis – being able to make sexual expression either exhilarating or debilitating.

Whilst it is not obvious to the naked eye, the pelvic floor can dictate a person's health and wellbeing. In addition, confidence and self-esteem are directly affected by the strength and condition of this hidden gem. The pelvic floor, unquestionably, works hard as the torso's foundation, but if that foundation fails to support or protect, then the consequences can be devastating. Like two ends of the spectrum, the pelvic floor is a subconscious measure of confidence when it is working efficiently, yet a conscious measure of a loss of that same confidence if/when dysfunction becomes a reality. Isolation, depression and a sense of hopelessness are all common feelings expressed as a result of problems associated with a pelvic floor that no longer works as it should. These problems include incontinence, pelvic organ prolapse (bladder, rectum, uterus or vaginal), vaginal dryness, laxity and/or atrophy, as well as erectile dysfunction. Any of these dysfunctions can lead to sex becoming far from sexy!

Furthermore, problems with the pelvic floor can have a detrimental effect on basic activities and experiences such as:

◆ Sports and/or exercise
◆ Lifting, pushing, pulling, twisting, jumping
◆ Laughing, coughing, sneezing
◆ Childbirth
◆ Sexual pleasure
◆ Menopause

Sexual satisfaction and continence are just two of the rewards for understanding the importance of and being responsible with your pelvic floor, and thus should be great motivators for maintaining its health. By understanding the basic role and duties of the pelvic floor, as a platform with the same responsibility for both sexes, you can save yourself from experiencing any of the above symptoms. Do not wait to suffer from one of the many dysfunctions that can afflict this poorly understood muscle group before you seek the education that empowers you to be in control at ALL times. Levity with regard to your pelvic floor could become very costly!

The Physical Pension Plan Investment Program - P3 is my parent company that I trademarked in July 2010 - Health & Finance in Harmony. Pelvic Floor Secrets is an integral part of that investment program that 'insures' retirement is about exploration, excitement and discovery, over pain and embarrassment. Your continued investment financially ensures that you are able to enjoy retirement with optimal health!

As the pelvic floor is impacted in our everyday movements, it is important to ensure its effectiveness to perform its role at all times, throughout our everyday lives and as such an awareness of its roles and responsibilities is essential, well before retirement age. Pelvic Floor Secrets is a reference bible for women (and men) from 20 to 120 years of age; the manual for pelvic floor practices that will ensure vaginal and pelvic floor health through sensory awakening, dietary adjustments and corrective exercise, with the ultimate conditioning assistance. It is enlightening, educational, entertaining and user friendly, with an elegance of language carefully balanced between science and colloquialism. Prepare to be empowered and sexy! Try the program and within as little as six weeks (provided you follow ALL of the instructions) you can begin to enjoy the success that it brings! If you never thought your confidence depends on it, think again!

Protect, Support, Satisfy and Stay Dry!
Enjoy xx

Better Sex!

WHENEVER I ask women which one of the following subjects they want to discuss first; Better Sex or Flatter Abs? The answer is always the same; better sex. This is the case regardless of culture or social status. The 21st century woman is very aware that her sexuality and sexual satisfaction plays an important part in defining who she is, how she is viewed and what she is advertising. Her body and body language truly are her adverts.

Today's female has a new confidence about her intimate encounters and wants to know that she is in control of the sensations that are experienced by both herself and her husband/partner. She wants to know that she can grip, massage and increase the sensations felt during orgasm. She is definitely an active part of the action! It does not matter how pretty she makes the outside – a 'vajazzle' will not be the lasting impression if, on the inside, she does not feel equally as great. Please note that whilst this book has a definite slant towards females, there is a chapter for the men, so be assured that men, I definitely have not forgotten you!

Chapter One

Better sex is empowering, it is commanding and it is rewarding. It is an amazing negotiator, a crazy end to a crazy night out, and the difference between a good relationship and its longevity. Whilst sex remains a relatively taboo subject in England in terms of discussion, the act of sex and the pleasure it can bring sits high on the agenda as the number one exercise to 'get Britain moving.' It requires no special clothing or footwear and no gym membership, just the confidence to strip bare in front of one other person (in most cases!).

Sex has become the focal point of many people's lives and relationships today. To have 'Better Sex' is a desire that more and more women are working towards and most men will go to amazing lengths to get.

Though an amazing pastime, hobby, and even a job or chore for the minority, sex can also be very judgemental. It is a great measure of confidence, overall wellbeing and ability. Typically, great sex is measured in a female by the tautness of her vagina, her agility and her willingness to be adventurous, as well as her endurance and sensitivity. In a man it is measured by the size of his manhood, his agility, his staying power, sensitivity and his selflessness. Whilst selflessness is important for both parties, it is the man's ability to delay ejaculation and ensure that his partner is fully satisfied before the encounter is over, that 'qualifies' him as a good and attentive lover.

Better sex is achievable by improving our ability to perform well. Our performance is determined by our flexibility, ingenuity, longevity and tautness, and these elements are directly affected by one set of muscles that are continually overlooked and rarely thought about

> " Sex has become the focal point of many people's lives and relationships today. To have 'Better Sex' is a desire that more and more women are working towards and most men will go to amazing lengths to get. "

> **"** *If I offered you £10,000 to clean my house – before you could enjoy the money, you would have to do the work. This is the same for the pelvic floor: in order for you to enjoy the reward, you have to (condition) do the work.* **"**

– the pelvic floor. Better Sex is the reward, it is NOT the primary purpose or responsibility of the pelvic floor.

If I offered you £10,000 to clean my house – before you could enjoy the money, you would have to do the work. This is the same for the pelvic floor: in order for you to enjoy the reward, you have to (condition) do the work.

The pelvic floor is a woman's secret weapon – her literal platform for success. It supports, protects and enhances her sexual expressions and experiences. It is a muscular sling that runs through the vaginal canal (with the upper part of the vagina sitting on it) and, as a muscle, it can be conditioned and strengthened. It is this muscular platform that responds during penetration and contracts extensively, if conditioned, during orgasm to increase the intensity and length of that sensation. This orgasmic explosion is a much nicer experience for both partners, and one which leaves the sexually satisfied woman with a distinct spring in her step.

In March 2011 I held a seminar series, which complemented the launch of my pelvic floor clinic in Central London. After one workshop session, whilst we were enjoying refreshments, a lovely lady came and very openly shared something very poignant with the entire group, which consisted of both males and females. She announced, "I love my vagina! I love the pleasure and joy it brings me, the way it pleases my husband, the way it makes me feel, it is amazing!" This should be the level of passion that every woman feels about her vagina.

For many years I have worked to create what my dear late friend Annette and I nicknamed "pin-head posse status", with the ultimate goal for this to be present, sensing and feeling. Towards the end of my first book, *Can a Vagina Really Buy a Mercedes?* I describe a cotton bud test, arguing that if you can grip a cotton bud with your vagina, then size is not the primary issue. However, I not only want to grip, I want to be able to massage and enhance the pleasure that we both feel from my actions. It really can bring about some amazing orgasms and makes for an insatiable appetite. I love it! Where I am able to win is through my awareness of and ability to coordinate my pelvic floor, which is conditioned, and combining this with the Swiss ball training that I have made a central part of my training program, makes for a very agile and flexible lower body. Being aware of how your body moves in space can make sex far sexier, intense and insatiably enjoyable.

Bringing Sexy Back!

When I was in hospital in 1994, about to give birth to my son, I jokingly said that I would, "Give Mother Nature a helping hand, just in case she forgot me." I began to do my pelvic floor exercises in my bed the very next morning. Whilst I did experience the pains of labour once my waters broke, I was still able to use the toilet, not the bedpan, and although I wanted and started to have a water birth, I actually found the water too cold and opted to go back to the bed, where I SLEPT before eventually being woken up to push. I remember my midwife commenting on how good I was during my labour with my breathing and pushing, and I thank my friend for the throwaway comment he had made a few years earlier, "My God, Jen, now I know what they mean when they say it's like dipping your wick in a well." His comment, my vanity and the will to do something about it, so no man would ever say that about me, saved my pelvic floor from dysfunction and ensured that I would have the taut vagina that his comment brought to my attention.

Imagine if you could package pelvic floor exercises as an Alexander McQueen dress; the biggest magazines would be ringing my phone off the hook. The Duchess of Cambridge would be my endorsement by default, and there wouldn't be enough hours in the day to handle the response. But unfortunately pelvic floor exercises are not tangible (although they are sexually, if managed well). And with these exercises, as with the pelvic floor itself, being neither seen nor thought about by the majority, only a select few will have taken the time to understand the benefits of the exercises and appreciate the speed at which results can be realised.

Think about the significance of the act of making love. It is the most significant practical application of the unification of two people. So significant is this act that a whole marriage ceremony and signing of the marriage register can be annulled if this act, the act of consummation, is not carried out on the first night. Sex in its raw form can be the most pleasurable thing for some women and the most tragic act for those who experience it because of abuse; and it is the legal requirement to confirm or seal a marriage. With this in mind, maybe we should not be quite so blasé about such an expression, but understand it, respect it and allow it to reward us accordingly.

Va-va-voom your vagina: become confidently continent and sexually satisfied. These are just some of the amazing rewards that can be achieved in as little as six weeks, by conditioning this most precious part of a woman's body.

1

In France, sexual satisfaction is very much recognised and worked towards inside a marriage, and the women there are generally very aware of their sexuality and the importance of pleasurable expression that is enjoyed by both partners.

It is also a mandatory requirement for women in France to undertake ten physiotherapy sessions after childbirth, in order to recondition the pelvic floor.

> *It is also a mandatory requirement for women in France to undertake ten physiotherapy sessions after childbirth, in order to recondition the pelvic floor.*

This ensures that vaginal laxity is not their destiny and that neither are continence pads! They are not embarrassed to work on the health of their pelvic floor – indeed, their proclivity to maintain the strength and condition of their most precious gift, allows them to continue to enjoy its rewards. These women are very much confidently continent and sexually satisfied.

London is the most cosmopolitan capital city in the world, and as a London girl myself, I get to enjoy the many museums and public parks in the city, as well as accessing some of the most amazing private health clubs and much improved public health centres. Personal training studios are opening up in all manner of places, and as such, access to health has never been so easy. But if you look around you on the underground and as you cruise in and out of the shops and shopping centres, you would not believe we have these facilities in such abundance. As a country we claim we are ahead of the game and yet English women top the European obesity charts (European Commission report, Nov 26, 2011) at 23.9% compared with just fewer than 22% of men. The European Commission recorded that nearly a quarter of British women were obese (16.6% in the 18-24 year age bracket), compared to their French or Italian counterparts – 12.7% and 9.3% respectively (figures based on a survey in 2008-2009, amongst the 19 European member states). I would love to be able to access the statistics for incontinence care and its increase at this time in order to identify a correlation.

As a nation we are celebrity driven and image aware, or body conscious, but that consciousness does not seem to extend to what the eye cannot see! Trust me, the statement, "What the eye can't see the heart cannot grieve about," does NOT apply to vaginal canals! If you are so willing to look good, why not ensure you feel good – down there as well? As one of my male friends told me for the first book, "We do not realise we are sitting on a gold mine!" I do not mean to be crass – I am simply stating a fact. And recently (Nov, 2011), at a networking event in Central London, a female solicitor said she had been told, "You have the P***Y you have the control!" A vulgar and quite disgusting statement I know, but these two statements give a brief insight into some of the conversations men have on the subject. They either discuss their sexual encounters with amazement or reluctantly divulge their bad experiences. Unfortunately, it is the bad experiences that are always remembered and think about it ladies, nobody continues to enjoy or return to a bad experience. We are and want to be recognised as the global hub of the world, so let us make sure we bring sexy back, not just sex! A recent study by Indiana University (published March 2012) showed that working our 'core' muscles along with our quads and inner thighs can help increase orgasms during sex after a workout, or indeed bring us to orgasm during our workouts! This is true, but only for those whose pelvic floor has a level of conditioning, and since the pelvic floor is the "core of the core," the more conditioned it is, the more likely the experience.

The de-conditioned female pelvic floor cannot grip, protect or support. It cannot contribute to orgasm, indeed the more laxity the less likely one will be able to orgasm.

Orgasms are described as an intense discharge of sexual tension in response to increased sexual activity that creates rhythmic involuntary contractions and increased sexual pleasure, euphoria. This sensation of better sex is not available to women whose pelvic floor strength and conditioning has been continually ignored, and as many researchers argue against Sigmund Freud's original finding in 1905 that orgasm was a direct response to penile, vaginal connection, it could be argued that his subjects had good pelvic floor conditioning that allowed them to experience these amazing vaginal orgasms without first stimulating the clitoris.

> The de-conditioned female pelvic floor cannot grip, protect or support. It cannot contribute to orgasm, indeed the more laxity the less likely one will be able to orgasm.

Whilst there are many women who have never experienced vaginal orgasm during penetration, it is hard to determine whether firstly, these women paid any particular attention to the contour and condition of their pelvic floor and vaginal canal, and secondly, whether they have co-ordinated the contractions into their intimacy and are able to disassociate the lower and upper body to increase the position of the penis along the 'roof' of the vagina where the clitoral "legs" run, thus increasing the likelihood for such an experience.

Better sex can help to keep us youthful, motivated and in healthier relationships.

Better sex can improve our aesthetics, confidence and overall wellbeing and better sex can elevate confidence exponentially!

Better sex can improve our aesthetics, confidence and overall wellbeing and better sex can elevate confidence exponentially!

As you read through this book and look at the diagrams, you will see just how complex this set of muscles really are. The pelvic floor is a junction: the link to the inner and outer world – letting passion in, and delivering life out! It is the gateway for elimination and pleasure. The pelvic floor gives way to life but can also give way to our organs, if its strength is not maintained. This most beautiful set of muscles sit within a gateway/junction that support the trunk from above and plays a major role in the function and movement of the legs which attach from below. If you never thought about or considered the importance of this gateway, the most precious part of our bodies, I hope this book will enlighten you. Your confidence and aesthetics, including posture and sexual expression, depend on it. Nothing in life is rewarding if it is not worked towards and better sex is no different. The pelvic floor works in exactly the same way in both males and females. The only difference is in the identification to activate it.

Invest Today, Enjoy Tomorrow

If we spend a little time conditioning and strengthening our vaginal walls and pelvic floor, we functionally narrow the vaginal diameter enabling us to massage our partners and increase the intensity of our

One of my success stories in this respect is Rianna. She came to one of my training classes initially to get healthy, but found the pelvic floor section the most exciting and paid special attention to ensuring she maximised her sensory pathways. Her husband paid attention also and the end result is a couple that are insatiable, excited and in tune with their bodies to the point of being able to grip and massage intensely. Her orgasms are explosive and mind-blowing and he is able to not only offset ejaculation, but to continue with an erection afterwards. They are a unique couple that have taken their intimate relationship to an amazing level.

orgasms. Functionally we are conditioning our pelvic floor through pleasure and we can literally bring our partners to a more powerful orgasm, functionally conditioning his prostate too. What a win-win all around. Lastly, for those of us worried about our body image, awakening the sensory pathways to the pelvic floor and then using the Gyneflex™ as a strength aid, not only improves the pelvic floor contour, but also improves the contour of the lower abdominal structure.

The beauty of this book is that it offers more than hope. It offers insight, empowerment, a positive outcome to ANY woman, wishing to realise her FULL female potential. It digs a lot deeper than the first book, taking a more in-depth look at the science and anatomy of the pelvic floor. This detail is necessary if we are to fully understand why we must look after the pelvic floor and if we are to allow ourselves the continued enjoyment of its many rewards. This book includes testimonies, diet advice, humour and candid insight. Once again, the language is user friendly and the resources needed to optimise your health have been made accessible. Use Pelvic Floor Secrets and Va-va-voom your vagina, from today.

Flatter Abs

MANY things can be used to judge the female figure, but one of the most poignant is the size and shape of her tummy; or more specifically the lower half. The lower abdominals are that part of the body that many women struggle with. A million crunches and still a pouch! Again, whoever told you that in order to look 'ABSolutely' fabulous, you should wrench your neck a thousand times, sold you a myth. The lower abdominals along with the pelvic floor, multifidus (true stabiliser of the lower back) and the respiratory

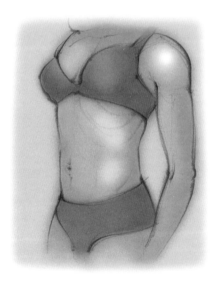

diaphragm, make up the 'core' of the trunk and these are the muscles that help to flatten the tummy. Think about it – if you condition everything above the belly button, why would the lower part look contoured, or function well? Another point to note is that this dreaded pouch that can establish itself below our belly buttons may not be there just as a result of excessive eating and lack of exercise, but as a result of a condition known as Visceroptosis.

Visceroptosis: when the organs of the viscera drop/fall from their anatomical position within the body. It is more prevalent amongst females and is the result of our body's dysfunctional natural girdle, which is made up of the transverse abdominals, obliques, multifidus, pelvic platform (floor), and quadratus lamborum. When these muscles do not work optimally, especially the transverse abdominals, they do not provide adequate support to hold the internal organs in their anatomical position, kidneys, liver, stomach and the colon begin to droop. This will place increased pressure on the digestive tract, uterus and bladder. Constipation can make the large intestine heavy and may also be a reason for the 'droop', and together this condition can lead to increased menstrual pain, incontinence and even pelvic organ prolapse as the picture shows: the uterus shifted downward towards the vaginal canal – first stage organ prolapse. (see page 26). (Reference: *How to Eat, Move & be Healthy*, Paul Chek, 2004).

Constipation is not a nice condition and should not be tolerated as a long-term condition for anyone. Optimal bowel movements should happen within 30 minutes to an hour after every meal. Going to the toilet every few days or once a week and even less is unhealthy. The toxic build up within the body is not good for long-term health, especially of the colon, which can be detrimental to it. The severity of constipation and its effect on the shape of the lower abdominals and pelvic floor are rarely explored and thus never really appreciated as a detrimental long-term contributor to pelvic floor problems or as one of the contributory factors to the dreaded pouch we fight so hard to get rid of. Constipation puts excess load on the large intestines, which in turn puts pressure on the lower abdominal wall and the pelvic floor. Without the correct lower abdominal/transverse (TVA) training – inner unit workout – the lower abdominals are not able to support the organs that 'sit' behind it effectively, and this leads

> " The severity of constipation and its effect on the shape of the lower abdominals and pelvic floor are rarely explored and thus never really appreciated as a detrimental long-term contributor to pelvic floor problems,... "

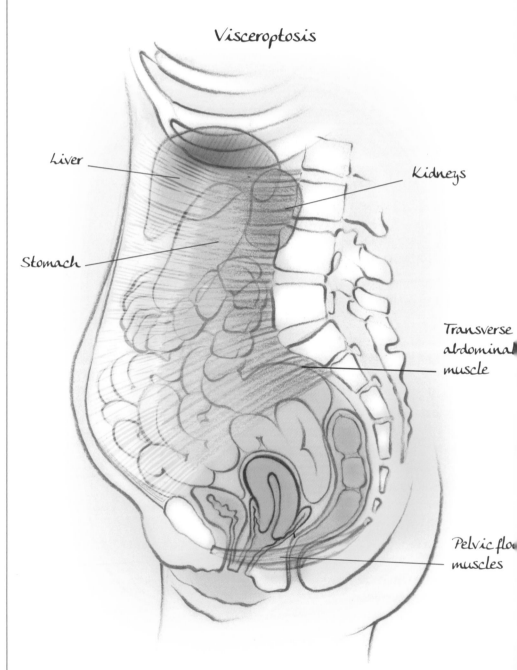

Visceroptosis

Liver

Kidneys

Stomach

Transverse abdominal muscle

Pelvic floor muscles

2

to the drooping mentioned in the paragraph above. Also, long-term constipation not only puts pressure on the pelvic floor in terms of load but also stresses the internal and external anal sphincters (described earlier under what is the pelvic floor), which can weaken their ability to close enough to prevent faecal incontinence.

What you eat and how much water you drink is crucial for good bowel habits, and good bowel habits are crucial to the maintenance of good pelvic floor health, functional lower abdominals and their aesthetics. The best way to empty the bowels is to squat on the floor above toilet tissue. Yes – not seated on the toilet. This is the ideal position, when the thighs are flexed against the abdomen the capacity of the abdominal cavity is lessened whilst intra-abdominal pressure is increased, encouraging expulsion. In this way, the position of the rectum is correct, unlike on the toilet seat where it is not fully relaxed. The squat position that the native Indians still use over a hole in the ground, allows for the following:

◆ Prevents 'faecal stagnation' – relaxation of the puborectalis muscle is achieved in this position, (where it would otherwise 'choke' the rectum whilst seated on the toilet) thereby allowing for total emptying of the colon contents
◆ Protection of the nerves that control the prostate, bladder and uterus, preventing them from becoming stretched and damaged
◆ Use of the thighs to support the colon and prevent straining, thereby taking pressure off the pelvic floor
◆ For pregnant women, it avoids putting pressure on the uterus when using the toilet and can help the mother prepare for delivery

◆ Securely sealing the ileocecal valve. The primary function of this valve is to limit the reflux of colonic contents into the ileum, which is the bottom part of the small intestine. The conventional sitting position can leave the valve unsupported and it can often leak during evacuation, which can contaminate the small intestine. (Reference: Jonathon Isbit, *Nature's Platform*)

If you are not so happy to squat on the floor then you should ensure you have a reasonably high stool in the bathroom that allows you to 'almost' replicate the position on the toilet. I have got many of my clients going to the toilet this way and funnily enough it is an invigorating way to go, and you do feel totally empty afterwards. The other lovely point is the abdominal wall will always appear flatter after. No do-do left; not full of it, not storing it, not carrying it around; awesome. (Jonathon Isbit, *Nature's Platform*).

A POINT TO NOTE: THE ILEOCECAL VALVE IS A SPHINCTER MUSCLE FOUND WHERE THE SMALL INTESTINE CONNECTS TO THE LARGE INTESTINE. IT IS LOCATED JUST ABOVE THE APPENDIX IN THE LOWER RIGHT SIDE OF THE ABDOMEN. WHEN THIS VALVE DOES NOT FUNCTION OPTIMALLY, GASTROINTESTINAL PROBLEMS, HEART SYMPTOMS, BLOOD PRESSURE PROBLEMS AND EVEN MIGRAINES CAN RESULT. MASSAGE CAN HELP TO ENCOURAGE PROPER FUNCTION.

> " *Flatter abs is not just achieved purely by exercise. Indeed, whether you like it or not, flatter abs are achieved by something we have all begun to abuse… food.* "

Flatter abs is not just achieved purely by exercise. Indeed, whether you like it or not, flatter abs are achieved by something we have all begun to abuse…food.

I remember attending a FirPro convention in 2000, where Paul Chek was giving a lecture on "How to flatten your abs forever!" I love this man, it has to be said, especially the way he teaches - dry and blunt. His knowledge of the spindle cells and the whole kinesiology of the body are phenomenal. Anyway, it was his first year at the convention and he caused contention. Maybe seen as arrogant, this man confidently stood on his word and brought a complete new perspective to exercise and exercise prescription, particularly of the trunk. His lecture on this one topic, which everybody wanted to master, was packed. The stairs of the auditorium became seats as the personal trainers in attendance thought they were about to learn the cutting edge exercise that would elevate them above their peers in their health clubs.

How disappointed we all were when there was not one single exercise in the whole lecture. Instead the lecture was completely focussed on what we ate, how we ate and when we ate it, and it all made sense. We love the food we eat, even if it bloats our stomach and causes excessive wind - it tastes good. Yet if we remove the fast food,

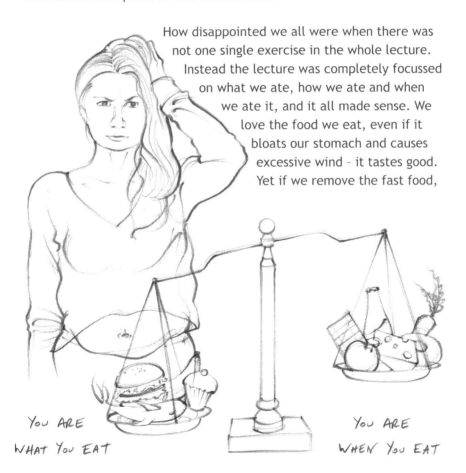

You ARE WHAT You EAT

You ARE WHEN You EAT

lager and wheat, we would shrink around our middle like it was going out of fashion. We would have a glow to our skin and have energy that would make us think we have been charged up like electricity. We would have learned that food was the source of that pouch that blights our skirts, trousers and dresses.

The lower abdominal, also known as the transverse abdominals, and pelvic floor are directly related. They are on the same neurological loop (fire wire to/from the brain). It is the synchronised activation of the lower abdominals with the pelvic floor that ensures full function. I say synchronised activation, because many people have no activation from their lower abdominals and therefore do not realise that they are not optimising the strength and condition of their pelvic floor simply because they are not using their body in the way it was designed to be used. The secret to effective pelvic floor training is to understand this correlation between the two and use them accordingly. Physiotherapists will tell you that you can work one in isolation of the other, but if they are working effectively one directly calls/pulls upon the other. The two share the same loop, along with the multifidus, which makes up the core – the body's natural stabiliser/weight belt – and therefore they work together to ensure stability of the trunk and support of the organs its contains. It just makes sense. The foundation of any structure, including our trunk, never works in isolation.

Flatter abs is another reward for being responsible with your pelvic floor, but exercise alone will not make them flat – SORRY. We do have to make adjustments to our eating habits if we are to win the war on the pot belly. Do not sigh too hard.

By eliminating or adjusting the portion size of our food, we can rid ourselves of the bloating that we may experience, especially after eating wheat based foods, as well as eliminating the gas – most unladylike, and this alone begins to shrink the tummy.

Next we need to establish what foods are good for the health of our pelvic floor and our libido and increase those, and lastly if we really want the flatter abs we crave and truly wish to experience great sex, then we need to understand the relationship between our diets and our expectations.

> 66 *By eliminating or adjusting the portion size of our food, we can rid ourselves of the bloating that we may experience, especially after eating wheat based foods, as well as eliminating the gas – most unladylike, and this alone begins to shrink the tummy.* 99

A POINT TO NOTE: Whilst the contour of
the lower abdominals can be improved, it is impossible to
measure the full function and see the full results if you
do not work on normalising your weight and optimising your
health by including an adjustment to your eating habits and
ensuring the right foods for your individual body makeup. The
Metabolic Typing® Diet will normalise your weight and thus
shrink the size of the pouch under the bellybutton, allowing you to
better ensure that it is not the obliques and rectus abdominals that
are indeed doing the work you think your lower abdominals are doing.

The shape of your bottom, your lower abdominal wall,
and the position of your knees and feet are a very
good indicator to a trained CHEK professional as
to whether the inner unit: pelvic floor, lower
abdominals, multifidus and respiratory
diaphragm are awake, synchronised and
working effectively. Most people can
experience flatter abdominals just be
eliminating wheat-based processed foods
such as white bread and many cereals that
actually have very little nutritional value.
We will take a look at food a little later.

2

Summary

In summary, flatter abs are a direct reflection of your good or bad gut health practices. It is important to understand that just as the gut is the foundation of your health, your stool is the evidence. Understanding the primary role food plays in your life and how it is reflected in your body's shape, texture of skin, as well as the whites of your eyes, hair, nails and teeth will always help you work toward a better outcome.

More than Technology

OUR bodies are the most amazing piece of kit on the planet. There is no technology in the world that can ever match it, FACT! The eleven systems that make up the body, the cells and hormones that regulate them, the "switch over" of a dominant system whenever another fails to work optimally – the adaptation of the body as we approach our mature years and begin to experience massive hormonal changes, especially in the area of reproduction – awesome.

Yet we take the mechanics for granted, not realising that although for many our health is 'given' to us at birth, we allow it to slip away by our lack of attention to/investment into how our bodies work. We do not read "the manual" so we have no idea how it all operates, just accepting and expecting the 'magic' that is the human body. When it begins to let us down however, we search for a solution, usually outside of ourselves, asking other, so called professionals, if they know the reason why 'we' are not operating optimally.

> **Healthcare professionals definitely have a place and have taken the time to study the human body and body mechanics so they are best positioned to offer a generic solution for all bodies. But the problem is that each of us is wired differently.**

Healthcare professionals definitely have a place and have taken the time to study the human body and body mechanics so they are best positioned to offer a generic solution for all bodies. But the problem is that each of us is wired differently. My reaction to meats, carbohydrates, fats, sleep, stress, exercise, breathing, physiological and environmental factors are completely different to yours, even if we seem the same on the surface.

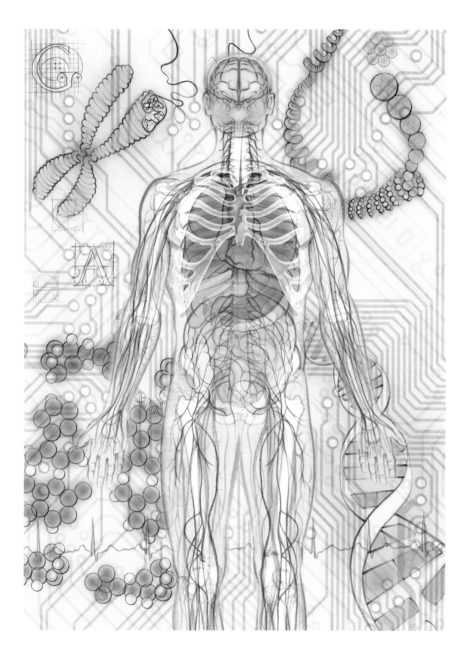

Chapter Three

My body can digest dark/dense meats really well and handle full fat desserts without the worry of excessive weight gain, constipation, headaches or bad skin, all of which are triggered by the body's reaction to the wrong food choices/plate portions. I have the energy to endure, although I no longer compete, I move and exercise, and thus make good use of the food I consume in the form of energy expenditure. Others, on the other hand, may eat the same foods as me and do the same things but may become constipated, feel lethargic and actually gain weight. It is the way in which our bodies use the food that we give it, which determines our health, body shape and overall wellbeing. It is no different to a petrol car being given diesel. It may move out of the garage and drive down the road but it will not go for long, and the mere fact that it managed to even move a little way on the wrong fuel, makes the damage and cost of repair much greater.

> " The function of our pelvic floor however, is exactly the same within all bodies: support, protection and satisfaction. "

The function of our pelvic floor however, is exactly the same within all bodies; support, protection and satisfaction. But whilst the function is the same the environmental and physiological factors are completely individual. It is crucial therefore for us to understand 'our' pelvic floor and to continue with a strength and conditioning program representative of an individual's lifestyle habits:

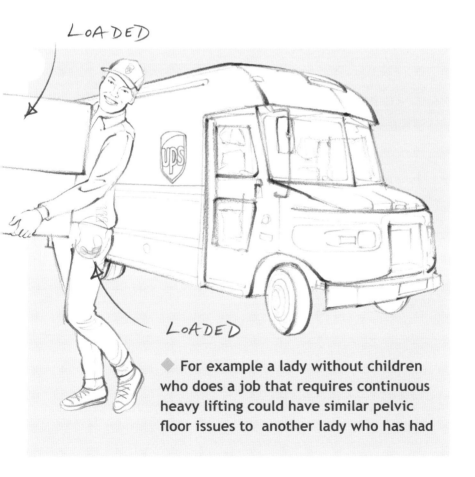

LoADED

LoADED

◆ For example a lady without children who does a job that requires continuous heavy lifting could have similar pelvic floor issues to another lady who has had

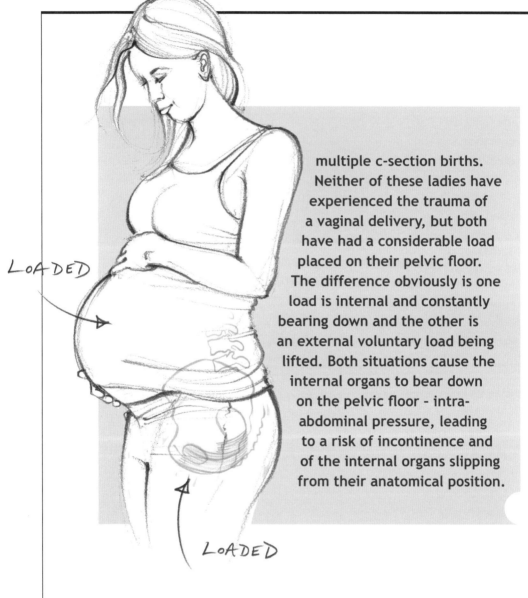

LOADED

LOADED

multiple c-section births. Neither of these ladies have experienced the trauma of a vaginal delivery, but both have had a considerable load placed on their pelvic floor. The difference obviously is one load is internal and constantly bearing down and the other is an external voluntary load being lifted. Both situations cause the internal organs to bear down on the pelvic floor - intra-abdominal pressure, leading to a risk of incontinence and of the internal organs slipping from their anatomical position.

In order to prevent these occurrences there must be good levels of high resting tone in the smooth muscles of the pelvic floor, confirming that the strength and condition of the pelvic floor is vital. Both situations also require protection of the lower back and good posture. It is a mistake to assume that a caesarean section means the pelvic floor is immune from dysfunction. If the babies are unusually heavy, or you have that load and are also continually lifting then there is an internal and an external load, and the forces downstairs could be major!

The lady with the caesarean section needs to be able to manage her load twenty four hours a day, seven days a week, whilst the lady who lifts needs to be able to manage the extra load she places into her hands during her working period. They both need to be able to squat effectively, but the types of squats they need to master could be totally different and thus impact their pelvic floor in a different way, but in a way that would offer maximum support when intra-abdominal pressure is increased (see later on in the book). If the women also hover over toilet seats or suffer from constipation then there is a downward force placed on the pelvic floor here also, one that could weaken it further over time.

The point is; no matter what the activity, we cannot escape loading this platform and therefore if we do not want to ever experience dysfunction, the best option is to acquire the education that will help to protect it and an appropriate strength and conditioning program, which does not consist of just stopping urine flow! Trust me; *'confident, continent, sexy and satisfied'* are four words you really will be able to use to describe yourself within.

The secret to a good pelvic floor is to investigate and understand its role and responsibility a little further than sex, and then to invest a little time and energy into the maintenance and upkeep, just like you would your car.

> " *The secret to a good pelvic floor is to investigate and understand its role and responsibility a little further than sex, and then to invest a little time and energy into the maintenance and upkeep, just like you would your car.* "

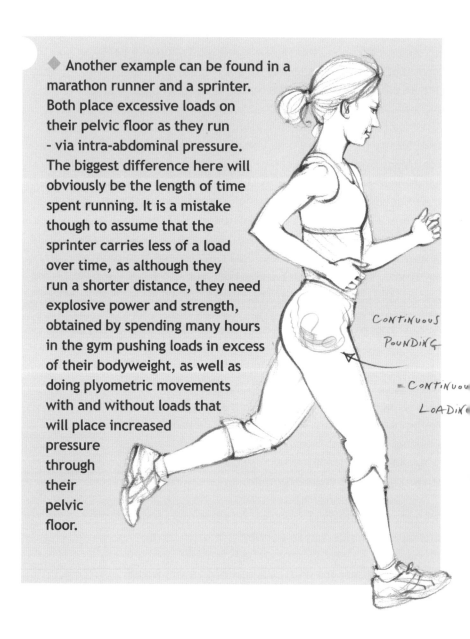

◆ Another example can be found in a marathon runner and a sprinter. Both place excessive loads on their pelvic floor as they run - via intra-abdominal pressure. The biggest difference here will obviously be the length of time spent running. It is a mistake though to assume that the sprinter carries less of a load over time, as although they run a shorter distance, they need explosive power and strength, obtained by spending many hours in the gym pushing loads in excess of their bodyweight, as well as doing plyometric movements with and without loads that will place increased pressure through their pelvic floor.

CONTINUOUS POUNDING

= CONTINUOUS LOADING

Since muscles cannot 'talk' they have to find another way to communicate their efficiency or deficiency! Fallen arches, valgus (knocked) knees, upright heart shaped bottoms (high and wide on the top) and the dreaded distended pouch in our lower abdominals, are all signs of a weakened pelvic floor or one that does not function as it should. It can also present as low back pain, knee pain and postural mis-alignment. This may be as a result of:

◆ Excess weight from fallen organs (viseroptosis see page 26).
◆ The smaller part of the glute max (big butt muscle) overworks when it finds itself 'having' to assist in the stability of the pelvis, instead of primarily focusing on extending the hip.
◆ Fallen arches and valgus knees usually go hand in hand as a result of overactive external rotators (piriformis, located within the pelvic basin) having to 'switch' from their primary role of rotating the hips to prevent our knees and feet from collapsing in, to assisting the glutes. They can also overwork as a result of trauma, injury, surgery and/or childbirth and their proximity to the sciatic nerve can cause many problems.

Figures can be as high as one in two women throughout the world, suffering some form of pelvic floor dysfunction: from a lack of sensation during intimacy to embarrassing "Oops" moments and/or prolapsed pelvic organs. A recent survey by Dr Hilary Jones on ITV's Lorraine morning show (October 2012) found that 84% of the women questioned had some form of incontinence with fewer than 40% seeking help from their GP due to the embarrassment and stigma attached to the subject. It is no wonder that when a group of women get together where three out of four have a dysfunction, you may find yourself singled out as the alien, if you are NOT suffering too. The misconception being that it is indeed a mandatory part of the ageing process!

We need to be able to place a real value in the role, responsibility, importance and REWARDS of our pelvic floor. Fortunately or otherwise, it is the effectiveness of the females' pelvic floor function and overall health, which determine:

◆ Her ability to "Get' and 'Remain' pregnant!

◆ Her ability to recover and recondition effectively after childbirth (especially natural), determine the strength of her sensations during intimacy, level of continence and thus her ability to enjoy the trampoline with her children and prevent pelvic organ prolapse.

◆ Her pelvic floor function, determines whether both partners enjoy the sensation in intimacy.

◆ Her pelvic floor function visible in her well shaped butt, lower abdominals and thighs as well as the natural arch in her feet (knees aligned), not only boosts her confidence, but increases the longevity of her health. All this keeps her pain and embarrassment free, insatiable and aesthetically pleased!

◆ Her pelvic floor dysfunction can make penetration painful and/or impossible.

Natural childbirth AND caesarean section do not have to be in exchange for full pelvic floor function, or diminished femininity.

A POINT TO NOTE: IT IS IMPORTANT TO UNDERSTAND THAT UNDERACTIVE (ATROPHIC) PUBOCOCCGYEUS MUSCLES WILL PRESENT AS "ROOMY" OR "VOID" WITHIN THE VAGINAL CANAL WHEN EXAMINED WITH THE INDEX FINGER, INSERTED AT THE SECOND JOINT (SOURCE: ARNOLD H. KEGEL, MD, FACS . STRESS INCONTINENCE AND GENITAL RELAXATION. CIBA CLINICAL SYMPOSIA, FEB-MAR 1952, VOL. 4, NO. 2, PAGES 35-52). WHEN THESE MUSCLES ARE

3

CONDITIONED AND WORK WELL THEIR ABILITY TO 'GRIP' OR 'CONTRACT' AROUND OR AGAINST THE
FINGER IS ACHIEVABLE FROM ALL THE WALLS OF THE VAGINAL CANAL.

Faulty recruitment of the pelvic floor muscles, which may be a result of childbirth, trauma, surgery or even faulty movement patterns (gait) can cause the ischiococcgyeus and piriformis muscles to become overactive (short and tight), whilst the pubococcgyeus (love muscles) become underactive (long and weak). This can not only lead to low back, and/or hip pain and urinary incontinence, but a lack of sensation and/or an inability to 'grip' during intimacy, making the experience less enjoyable. If this happens it is important to relax and 'switch off' the instant recruitment from the overactive ischiococcgyeus and piriformis muscles FIRST and then strengthen the sling, from the pubococcgyeus up in order to use the entire pelvic floor for improved aesthetics, support, protection and sexual function.

Since the piriformis 'sits' so close to the sciatic nerve, an adverse increase in its size and activation can compress the nerve causing numbness through the butt and down the leg on the side affected as well as low back pain. Whilst it is important to keep this muscle strong it must remain "Flexible".

It is a mistake to believe that ALL pelvic floor programming start with strength and conditioning! Sensory awareness must always be the starting point for ALL pelvic floor programmes, to avoid faulty recruitment of muscles such as the piriformis which can lead to long-term loss of sensation within the pelvic floor and vaginal canal.

What is the Pelvic Floor?

THE pelvic floor is the foundation of the trunk. In my opinion it is the most precious part of a woman's body (can directly affect a man's confidence and/or ego). It is the gateway that links our inner and outer worlds; assisting in the stability of the trunk and supporting the internal organs in their anatomical position within the trunk, eliminating waste (urine and faeces), bringing forth life and for many women enabling them to have the most amazing orgasms and sexual expression by enhancing the strength and/or condition of the vaginal canal.
The pelvic floor is an integral part of core stability. It assists in the proper positioning of a baby's head during childbirth and controls the flow of urine (continence). It is referred to as the love muscle because it plays an important part in 'gripping' your partner by contracting during orgasm, which increases the pleasure and experience.

For the lady who knows where and what her pelvic floor can do for her, it can be the start of something increasingly insatiable.

But for the lady who does not know or has paid no attention; pain and embarrassment may well be her portion, in place of pleasure.

> " For the lady who knows where and what her pelvic floor can do for her, it can be the start of something increasingly insatiable. "

The little example mentioned above shows just how the pelvic floor, in conjunction with the lower abdominals, 'saves' us from embarrassment, by elevating and ensuring our urethral and anal sphincters remain sealed shut during these seamlessly simple movements that

If you've never paid any real attention to the activity within your pelvic floor muscles:
- Place your hands on your tummy next time you laugh or sneeze and focus on how your abdominal wall responds.

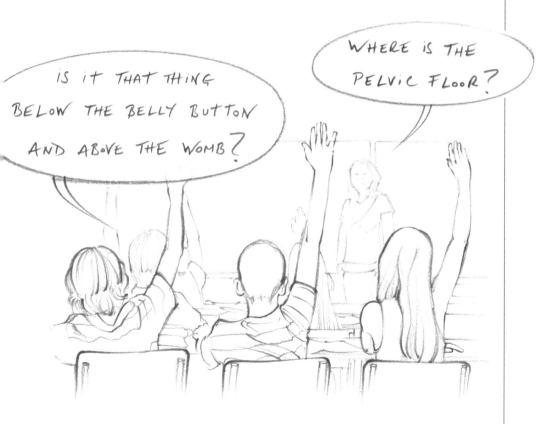

could otherwise have a different outcome. Both the resting tone and voluntary contractions are important for optimal pelvic floor support, as both of these determine continence when carrying out all activities.

When you carried out the above example you should have felt a little pulling inwards of your belly button and at the same time a little elevation from within the vagina or at least the perineum (that little area between the vagina/penis and the anus) and if you place your hand by your diaphragm it elevates too as your organs move.

Studies such as Christie & Colosi 2008, stated that one in three women has some form of pelvic floor dysfunction; incontinence, pelvic pain or pelvic organ prolapse. I meet women every day with one of these conditions, who feel a sense of hopelessness when an operation or continence pads are the only solution. Viktru, Rortveit & Lose 2006, stated that pregnancy is commonly associated with the start of pelvic core weakness, with many women also experiencing lower back pain (directly linked to pelvic floor dysfunction) and diastasis recti – a splitting of the abdominal muscles at the Linea Alba (middle of the abdominals) which can lead to the lower abdominal protrusion or "pooch" (as mentioned earlier) that so many women tend to develop after childbirth or significant weight loss.

The pelvic floor, transverse abdominals, respiratory diaphragm and the multifidus, make up the inner unit core. It is a synergistic working relationship coupled with a relationship with the hips and abductors, and receptors from the brain, which can be interrupted at any point along the spinal column by trigger points from the trunk. In my first book, 'Can a Vagina Really Buy a Mercedes?' I describe this unit as a can, with the base being the pelvic floor, the lid the diaphragm and the sidewalls as the support that keeps the two ends apart and the contents

Female Organs

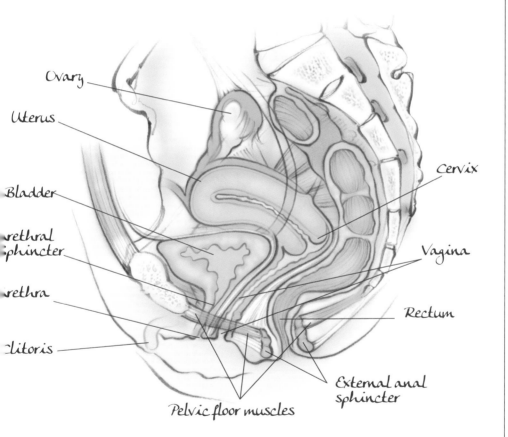

Ovary

Uterus

Bladder

Urethral sphincter

Urethra

Clitoris

Cervix

Vagina

Rectum

External anal sphincter

Pelvic floor muscles

in place. The inner unit, diet, weight, hydration, and poor exercise prescription can directly affect its strength and condition. This means that to focus on the pelvic floor in isolation of all these sets of muscles does not work towards optimal health. Indeed, posture plays a big part in pelvic floor function.

Every muscle is fed by sensory receptors from the brain and the pelvic floor is one of the "forgotten" receptors. We activate our muscles via sensory programming, but as this is a hidden muscle that works under 'subconscious' voluntary control when fully functional, we assume there is no need for this training. Alas, this thought process has caused much pain and embarrassment for many women (and men). Whilst it is controlled by sensory programming it is still a muscle with a huge responsibility and a lot of load continually placed on it, so to not strengthen it, is to leave it vulnerable and weak. Muscles that are short and tight need stretching and muscles that are weak and long need strengthening. The pelvic core muscles may also lose their reflexive capability to "turn on" automatically, providing support to the entire core from the bottom up. When this happens, a potential solution is three-dimensional core training that integrates the pelvic floor muscles and PCNS (Moen et al. 2007).

Just by the nature of its position and responsibility, coupled with the lifestyles we lead and the adverse load we continue to place on it when we run, jump, skip, twist, push, pull, lift, bend, sneeze, cough and laugh, we must consider embarking upon a pelvic floor strength and conditioning program.

> " Just by the nature of its position and responsibility, coupled with the lifestyles we lead and the adverse load we continue to place on it when we run, jump, skip, twist, push, pull, lift, bend, sneeze, cough and laugh, we must consider embarking upon a pelvic floor strength and conditioning program. "

The pelvic floor is the last sensory pathway to be awakened and usually one of the first to be trashed. When we potty train our children, we are teaching them to understand the sensation and urge to empty, and to link that to getting to the toilet and taking down their pants before they do so. It is a sensory program where the coordination/fire-wire from the brain to the pelvic floor is being synchronised. Little Johnny may like to empty his bowels at 9.22am every day, but at the age of four he starts school where break time is at 10.30am. For the first few days the teacher may entertain little Johnny's request, but soon she/he will ask Johnny to wait until break time. With the new instruction to wait until 10.30, Johnny's sphincter muscles are being reprogrammed to stay shut instead of relaxing for evacuation, and within 21 days this becomes a new automatic motor engram (message from the brain) and his body's position of strength. When he goes to sit on the toilet he now needs to strain to open his bowels because his brain has taught his muscles to stay shut instead of void and relax.

Indeed it is the best way to activate the Transverse Abdominals (TVA), and then once you have switched on this "lost sensory unit", you can condition it whilst working out or carrying out your everyday activities. This is how you become in control at ALL times in ALL activities.

Switching on the sensory pathways first, becoming acutely aware of closing the vaginal wall and elevating as well as relaxing (opening) and dropping, in sync with breathing, will begin to retract the transverse abdominals almost as if someone is physically pulling them from inside. Couple this with the Gyneflex™ and you can really begin to condition these muscles from the inside.

We carry this pattern on when we do not like the toilets that we use; where instead of them being a place where we eliminate waste in a relaxing environment, the experience becomes distressing. All of this is not good for our pelvic floor, which is not sure what it is now supposed to be doing. Constipation is a big thrasher of the pelvic floor. Now if little Johnny, who is now constantly constipated, then becomes obese he will increase his problems. This scenario is true for little girls too. With that in mind, it is a shame that toilets are not treated with the level of respect that allows us to relax and eliminate. After all, all waste is toxic, so to hold onto it can only become detrimental to our health over time. I met Sergute in 2010 when she came down from Birmingham to style me for an article to feature in a new magazine, Juno Lucina. It is amazing how you can impact a person just by sharing your information in an informal setting. As my stylist now, I have seen her many times, and although she is a lovely 25 years young, the information I have given her has registered and she has taken pleasure in sharing with her work colleagues. Here is an example of just one of those conversations, as told to me:

"One of my mates was complaining about the lack of action he was getting after his wife had their baby. Very quickly a colleague in her mid-forties jumped to his wife's defense and sparked a debate on a woman's healing process after giving birth. When I interjected that one of the main reasons why a woman's childbirth experience left the body in such shock was because the muscles of her pelvic floor were not conditioned or activated correctly for the purpose of childbirth, all five of the people in the conversation turned around and looked at me like I was a mad woman!

I began to explain that a woman needed to learn how to not only engage her pelvic floor muscles for childbirth, but more importantly relax them for delivery, the lady who was being sympathetic to the wife said, 'You don't know what you are talking about. You only do pelvic floor exercises once you've had the child in order to stop wetting yourself!'Everyone else was in agreement. I continued to tell them that the muscles should be trained just like any other muscle in the body, both before and after childbirth, because if they are in tune beforehand then less damage occurs to the pelvic floor and the healing process can be shorter. I could have been laughed right out of Birmingham with their reactions! The main view being that I was a silly little girl that did not know any better.

Personally, I could not believe how ignorant people are about the human body, treating the pelvic floor differently to their other muscles and not believing that the muscles require exercise or strengthening like the rest of our body. It was at that moment I thought, thank God for Jenni, because I could have been just as ignorant as them. Believe me I am making sure that I look after my pelvic floor muscles before and after I have my child, or children, so that I too can have a continued healthy sex life. Thank you, Jenni. You saved my confidence!"

This is a great example of how little people know and/or understand this hidden gem and one reason for this is because of the lack of information available.

Accessibility to information that advises us on how to strengthen our pelvic floor is only freely available to women after 'natural' childbirth, on a sheet of A4 paper that most mothers tend to misplace or throw away.

Its importance to their recovery and total health is as unimportant as the paper it is presented on, and the information on it has barely improved in recent years, 'almost allowing' dysfunction to continue to rise at alarming rates.

> **Accessibility to information that advises us on how to strengthen our pelvic floor is only freely available to women after 'natural' childbirth, on a sheet of A4 paper that most mothers tend to misplace or throw away.**

Firstly, the information provided is not always entirely appropriate, and secondly, it cuts out a whole society of women who have either had no children or have not experienced vaginal delivery, since it is still a common belief that the pelvic floor is affected only/primarily by this. Natural childbirth is the most amazing experience. Nothing can compare to it, and when you finally see the bundle of joy that you have been carrying around and then 'pushed out', it is unexplainable! It saddens me though to think that for the sake of a little care and attention - conditioning this amazing gateway, women are sacrificing this beautiful experience in order to save themselves from the embarrassment of pelvic floor dysfunction. What they are not understanding/realising, is that they can experience exactly that same embarrassment because of sport, age, surgery, weight and everyday movements, simply because they are unaware of the impact of these everyday stressors on the pelvic floor. If you do not believe me, ask a gynaecologist if they ever see women without children who have the 'Blackwall Tunnel' going on down there and wait for their response. Babies can make the pelvic floor weaker and expand the vagina, but so too can many other things!

The following science lesson is necessary, if only to give you a better insight into the complexity of the muscles that make up the pelvic floor and how their synchronicity allows our floor to work effectively. A valuable connection to understand is the fascial connection of the pelvic floor muscles (levator ani) to an important hip muscle (obturator internus) via the arcuate tendon. The pelvic floor muscles are also fascially connected to the adductors, which provide a balanced, equal and opposite reaction to the obturator internus. All of these interconnections produce chain reaction activation of the pelvic floor muscles when hip rotation moves are added to a core training exercise.

The pelvic floor is located at the base of the abdominal cavity and is made up of three main layers. (You can run your hand across the base of the abdominals just above your pubic bone to locate it). It spans across the opening within the bony pelvis, connecting to the pubic bone at the front and the coccyx at the back, forming a supporting layer for the abdominal and pelvic viscera (internal organs of the body, such as the intestines). The upper part of the vagina, urethra, bladder and supporting structures of the pelvis are all part of the pelvic floor. It is one of the most complex and poorly understood sets of muscles within the body; the junction and gateway that links the lower limbs and torso.

There are three main layers:

The first layer is the endopelvic fascia. It covers tightly around the bladder, the inner organs such as the intestines and the uterus in women, providing support. It is a mesh of smooth muscle fibres, ligaments, nerves, blood vessels and connective tissue. The collagen within the endopelvic fascia provides the strength needed to ensure the organs remain in their anatomical position. Some of these ligaments attach to the lumbar spine and the symphysis pubis. Although this layer cannot be exercised, the muscles in the second layer (pelvic diaphragm) can improve/offset any back pain by increasing the support they give to the bladder and uterus from below, decreasing the strain placed on the ligaments.

A POINT TO NOTE: IF A WOMAN WERE TO SUFFER A TEAR IN THE ENDOPELVIC FASCIA, FOR EXAMPLE, BECAUSE OF A DIFFICULT DELIVERY OR ANOTHER INJURY, THEN STRENGTHENING THE PELVIC FLOOR CAN HELP TO SUPPORT THE BLADDER, UTERUS AND RECTUM.

The second layer is the most talked about, and is of most significance for support and sexual function. The levator ani, "the lifter of the anus", is a hammock shaped, meshed sling, that supports the weight of the pelvic contents and acts to resist increased intra-abdominal pressure (pressure from inside the muscle) which comes about as a result of our everyday activities: bending over to pick up a heavy object, sneezing, laughing, coughing, running, jumping, pushing, pulling, twisting etcetera, with gravity adding its own natural pressure. The levator ani needs to guarantee continence at night and thus it has a high resting tone, which makes it completely different from other

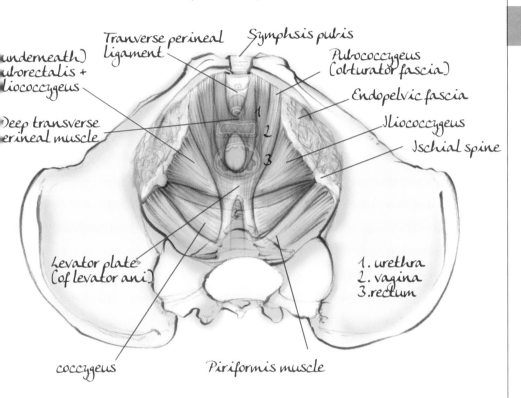

4

Female pelvis superior view

Tranverse perineal ligament

Symphsis pubis

(underneath) (ubrorectalis + Iliococcygeus

Pubococcygeus (obturator fascia)

Endopelvic fascia

Deep transverse erineal muscle

Iliococcygeus

Ischial spine

1
2
3

Levator plate (of levator ani)

1. urethra
2. vagina
3. rectum

coccygeus

Piriformis muscle

smooth skeletal muscle where the tone is far less. It is stimulated by the pudendal nerve (the nerve which feeds the signals to the perineum), which causes quick pre-contractions in order to ensure we maintain continence whenever we do any activities, including those mentioned above.

Within the levator ani are a series of muscles, which make up what is known as the pelvic diaphragm:

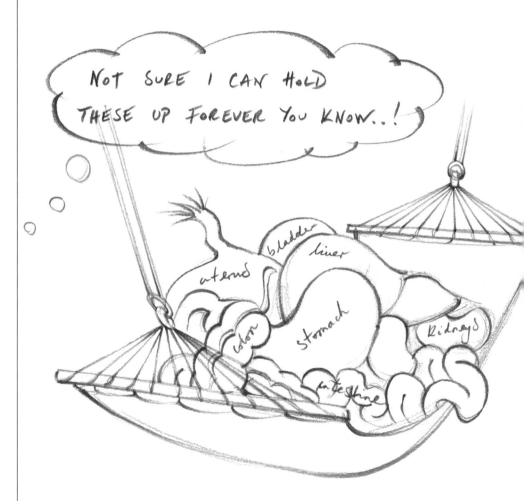

◆ The pubovisceral muscle, also known as the pubococcygeus, pulls the rectum, vagina and urethra forwards towards the pubic bones, compressing their lumens (openings). The pubococcygeus is a hammock-like muscle, which is part of the pelvic diaphragm and muscles that form the levator ani. It stretches from the pubic bone to the coccyx (tail bone), forming the floor of the pelvic cavity and supporting the pelvic organs. Increasing the strength of this muscle group would assist in increasing the closure of these structures and improve the 'grip' we women can have on our partners as well as the intensity of our orgasms.

◆ The puborectalis muscle loops around the rectum, pulling it forward during contraction and assisting in the provision of continence

◆ In women, the pubovaginalis muscle loops around the vagina, from front to back and

◆ In men, the levator prostatae muscle supports the prostate gland

◆ The iliococcygeus muscle extends from the tailbone to each of the sitting bones. Some of the fibres run side to side and some diagonally, but they are not involved in lifting the anus

◆ The coccygeus muscle lies next to the iliococcygeus muscle and can influence the stability of the sacroiliac joint. Any abnormal tension of this muscle can keep the sacroiliac joint in a displaced position and cause pain that can run into the hamstring.

The third layer is the urogenital diaphragm. It is the outermost layer of the pelvic floor and is made up of several muscles. The deep transverse perineal muscle is very important for ensuring continence and it supports the function of the levator ani. The other muscles of this layer are important for sexual function, even though they do not support the organs of the pelvis.

The sphincter of this muscle, the urogenital sphincter, loops around the urethra in both men and women, assisting with continence (urogenital concerns the organs of the urinary tract and the reproductive organs, when considered together. The sphincter is a circular band of muscle surrounding an opening or passing in the body, which narrows or closes the opening by contracting). Pelvic floor exercises can increase the strength of the urogenital sphincter, which is a striated muscle under some voluntary control:

◆ The bulbocavernosus muscle connects the bulb of the penis to the urogenital diaphragm, causing it to contract during ejaculation or at the end of urination. In women it contracts during orgasm, erecting the clitoris. The fibres of this muscle run from front to back

◆ The ischiocavernous muscle increases the erection in men and erects the clitoris in women. Its fibres run in a diagonal direction

◆ The anal sphincter muscles loop around the anus like a ring and provide continence of the rectum. Along with the puborectalis, the external anal sphincter works together to close the anal canal. 80% of the resting tone is involuntary (works naturally) and 20% is under voluntary control, for example to stop the passing of wind

Forceps, tears and/or an episiotomy can occasionally damage the sphincters.

Female pelvis medial view

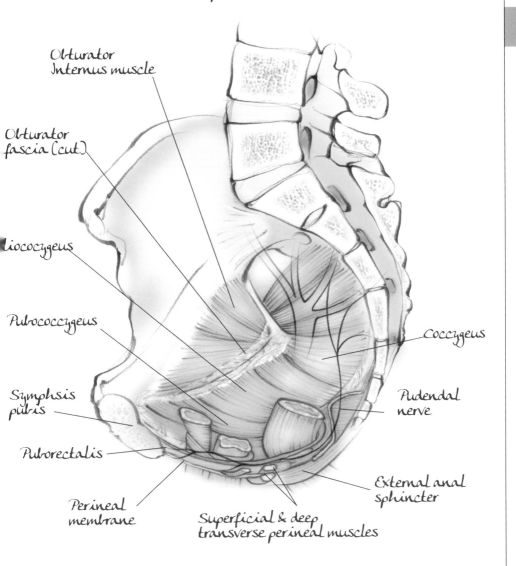

Obturator
Internus muscle

Obturator
fascia (cut)

Iliococcygeus

Pubococcygeus

Symphsis
pubis

Puborectalis

Perineal
membrane

Superficial & deep
transverse perineal muscles

Coccygeus

Pudendal
nerve

External anal
sphincter

◆ Hormonal changes such as the menopause, which results in a loss of estrogen, can weaken the pelvic floor structures causing urinary leaks and/or pelvic organ prolapse, as can aging

The symphysis pubis is not a layer of the pelvic floor, although it is crucial to understand its role, especially for new mums to be. It is a very small cartilaginous joint (a joint made up entirely of cartilage that allows movement between bones) that sits in the midline of the left and right pubic bones. It attaches to the vulva in females, intimately close to the clitoris, whilst attaching above the penis in males, with the sensory ligament of the penis attaching to the symphysis pubis. It is roughly 2mm wide with a one degree rotation and this increases for women at the time of childbirth. The gracilis is a slender superficial muscle of the thigh that attaches to the lower half of the symphysis pubis and the upper half of the pubic arch, as do hip adductors. These are all attached to the posterior side of the femur and thus when dysfunction occurs in the symphisis pubis joint, any lateral movement can cause excessive pain. Joint stability is crucial during pregnancy; it is reported that up to 25% of women find the symphisis pubis to be the cause of much pain as a result of the hormone relaxin making the whole joint unstable. It is important then to understand the increased flexibility that is available during pregnancy because of the presence of relaxin and subsequently to endeavour not to overstretch. Diastasis of the symphysis pubis, which is literally a dislocation without a fracture, is the separation of the two bones, causing pelvic girdle pain. This affects approximately 45% of pregnant woman and 25% of postpartum women. Symphysis pubis dysfunction is another symptom of pelvic girdle pain again caused by excessive movement of the pubic bones, which can cause a misalignment. It is important

> *Whilst flexibility is important, you do not want to weaken muscles or even ligaments and tendons by overdoing it in classes like Yoga or Pilates.*

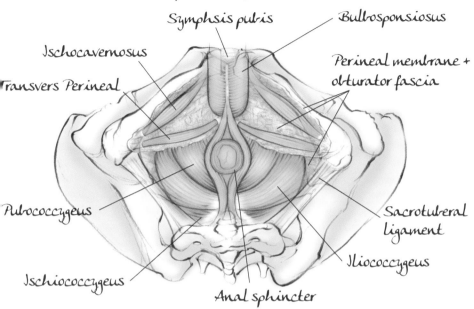

Female pelvis inferior view

Symphsis pubis

Bulbosponsiosus

Ischocavernosus

Perineal membrane + obturator fascia

Transvers Perineal

Pubococcygeus

Sacrotuberal ligament

Ischiococcygeus

Iliococcygeus

Anal sphincter

to seek advice from a specialist therapist who can prescribe corrective exercise to enhance the stability of the pelvic girdle.

A POINT TO NOTE: THE BODY BECOMES DYSFUNCTIONAL WHEN MUSCLES ARE EITHER SHORT AND TIGHT OR LONG AND WEAK. RELAXIN CAN BE 'MISUSED' TO INCREASE FLEXIBILITY AND RANGE OF MOVEMENT, WHICH CAN BE DETRIMENTAL TO THE PELVIC GIRDLE IF NOT RECOGNISED.

Whilst flexibility is important, you do not want to weaken muscles or even ligaments and tendons by overdoing it in classes like Yoga or Pilates.

Be aware of and control or limit your range of movement during pregnancy.

"If little attention is paid to the importance and relevance of pelvic floor exercise especially during pregnancy and childbirth, then the experience during the delivery can cause otherwise avoidable damage to the female and be very traumatic for both the new mother and her husband who witnesses and hears the tear!"

Chris Heron, Founder Shaping Change.
www.shapingchange.co.uk

You will be surprised at how negatively pelvic floor dysfunction can impact on your relationship. Take charge, just as men have to take charge of their prostate. Flip the switch for a moment; erectile dysfunction is rising at an alarming rate and many doctors are not recognising the link between that and the added stress faced by modern man and the effect of his increasing girth, which decreases testosterone and increases estrogen levels. These hormone changes subsequently affect libido and a man's ability to sustain an erection.

Again, the drive for external gratis is a major contributor to the stress: the house, location, contents, gadgets, car, bank account, keeping kids in line with 'The Joneses' etcetera. His role of provision has taken over, almost to the detriment of protection, because our material expectations and desires are too high. We want to wait for nothing and we want the best of everything; everything that is except the best of health. Food is sourced cheaply to make way for the trappings of success, so the family is not feeding the body optimally. Bedtime is a luxury, as is relaxation, so adequate repair and restoration of the mind and body's systems, which happens when we sleep, is diminished. This is compounded with the male ego desiring a big chest and biceps. Men are lifting heavier loads: manually at work, at home and in the gym, without regard for their pelvic floor, which works in exactly the same way as ours. As they lift, there should be an elevation of the pelvic floor. This is felt through the testes and it is this that ensures support, not just of the organs, but also for the lower back when the transverse abdominal is activated. If the pelvic floor is bearing down, it is the contents of the trunk as well as the external load that is pushing on it, and over time it becomes weak. Do not become disempowered by your pelvic floor. It is truly the most powerful expression within your body.

Many men lift heavy loads and hold their breath, which causes even more pressure on the pelvic floor. The overdeveloped chest alters posture, pulling the chest down onto the diaphragm, restricting the airways and thus not allowing oxygen to flow freely to the lower part of the body. For both men and women, pelvic floor health is dependent on a good oxygen supply, so the respiratory diaphragm needs to remain open and fully functional.

Male pelvic floor dysfunction has such an impact on a man's ego, relationship, libido and self-esteem that he invariably seeks to find a solution much quicker than us ladies.

A young man is not going to just accept TENA for Men – no, he will want to know how to fix it and although the resources are limited, he will source them.

Everybody has a hang up they believe they can live with, but ladies it should not be incontinence, pelvic organ prolapse, vaginal laxity and/or dryness.

> " Male pelvic floor dysfunction has such an impact on a man's ego, relationship, libido and self-esteem that he invariably seeks to find a solution much quicker than us ladies. "

Va-Va-Voom your Vagina

Our vagina can be the gateway that provides endless hours of sexual pleasure and new life. It is the gateway for elimination and menstrual flow, but it can also be the gateway for prolapsed pelvic organs and embarrassing incontinent 'Oops' moments. To consider a pelvic floor conditioning program, whilst overlooking the role the muscles within the vaginal canal play to assist in protecting and preventing dysfunction, could be detrimental in the long run.

Indeed the 100 trillion bacteria that live within the vaginal canal and their importance and relevance to the health of the baby as its first line of defence as it passes through, which help to strengthen the baby's immune system, is reason enough to ensure vaginal health and hygiene.

> " *A little bit of conditioning, even as little as three times per week for 10-15 minutes, is all that is needed to ensure that the whole world and his uncle cannot get inside there and start playing football!.* "

Unfortunately, the vagina is seen primarily as an object of sexual pleasure with no regard to how it lives within the pelvic floor, and how its condition or de-condition can contribute to either support and protection or total prolapse that can fall right through to the outside world where it becomes visible, and the affected organ exposed to infections including recurring urinary tract infections (UTIs) which can be very painful.

Va-va-voom your vagina from today; 'Be Ready, Be Educated' and do not let it be the brunt of any man's jokes when he gets together with his friends to discuss the abyss you could end up having down there.

Chapter Five

The muscles of our vaginal wall contract, relax and expand, alongside the pelvic floor. Our vaginal canal expands to "allow" the penis to enter the vagina, relax and expand to allow the baby along and through the vaginal canal, and contract with the help of the pelvic floor to "grip" our husbands or partners.

All muscles have memory and "our position of strength" is whatever or however we train these muscles to be, whether conscious or unconscious.

Repeated sexual expression with bigger and bigger objects, without a complimentary contraction program, can by default condition the vaginal canal to 'believe' its position of strength and/or 'natural' position is to be 'open.' The problem with this is that it 'helps' the pelvic floor and vaginal canal to 'register and keep' a position of laxity (looseness).

A functional conditioning program for pelvic floor and vaginal health must know how to contract and relax in a "split second"! The quicker the reaction times from these two positions and the 'stronger' the 'grip and elevation' the more functional and healthy the pelvic floor and the better protected and less likely an incontinent experience or prolapsed organ.

Ladies, a little bit of invested time into pelvic floor exercise today, can make life a lot sexier tomorrow! In order to continue to/or understand this most precious part of our body, let me now breakdown the vagina just as I did with your pelvic floor:

Vagina – 'elastic' muscular canal with a soft, flexible lining. It has a very high concentration of nerve endings that provides sensation when stimulated and self-lubricates when aroused. The vagina connects the uterus to the outside world, with the vulva and labia forming the entrance and the cervix of the uterus protruding into the vagina, which forms the interior end. It lies midway between the anal tract and the urethra. The entrance and length of the canal (retroverted {pointing backward} or normal) is usually 6 - 7.5 cm (2.5 - 3 in) across the anterior (front) wall and 9 cm (3.5 in) long across the posterior (back) wall. The elasticity and lubrication of the vagina allows it to stretch to accept the penis during intercourse, (and allow for natural childbirth) helping to reduce friction.

With arousal, the vagina lengthens rapidly to an average 10 cm (4 in), and can continue to lengthen in response to pressure placed upon it. As a woman becomes fully aroused, the last two thirds expand in length and width, whilst the cervix retracts.

Along the inside of the vulva, the walls of the vagina are a reddish pink colour, with soft elastic folds of mucous membrane which form ridges that stretch and contract. This movement is assisted by the pelvic floor muscles, allowing for stretching to the size of the inserted penis, stimulating the penis and helping to cause the man to experience orgasm (ejaculation), making fertilisation possible.

Bartholin's glands - vaginal lubrication is provided by the Bartholin's glands, which are located near the vaginal opening and the cervix. The membrane of the vaginal wall produces moisture, even though there are no glands within them. Before and during ovulation, the mucus glands of the cervix secrete different variations of mucus, which provides an alkaline environment in the vaginal canal that is favourable to the survival of sperm.

Vaginal shortening - can happen when pelvic surgery is performed, including hysterectomy and/or pelvic floor surgery such as vaginal repair of organ prolapse. The top of the vagina can scar downwards after a hysterectomy or the walls can scar together, affecting its elasticity and significantly shortening the vagina. This can lead to severe pain with intercourse, preventing deeper penetration or preventing intercourse altogether, depending on the severity of the shortening.

5

When a woman is standing, the vaginal tube points in an upward – backward direction, at an angle a little more than 45 degrees with her uterus. The vaginal opening is at the caudal (tail) end of the vulva, behind the opening of the urethra. The upper quarter of the vagina is separated from the rectum by the recto-uterine pouch (deepest point of the peritoneal cavity, behind the uterus and in front of the rectum).

The hymen - is a membrane of tissue, which is situated at the opening of the vagina. This may be ruptured during penetration, delivery, a pelvic examination, injury or sports. The absence of a hymen does not necessarily indicate prior sexual activity, as it is not always ruptured during sexual intercourse. Similarly, its presence does not always indicate a lack of previous sexual activity, as light activity may not rupture it either and it is possible to surgically restore it. It is the breaking/tearing of the hymen that is seen within the Bible as the blood covenant for marriage consummation.

Vestibular bulbs - The vestibular bulbs are located in the internal part of the clitoris. (They can also be found in the vestibule, the space between the labia

> 66 **Vaginal shortening**
> *- can happen when pelvic surgery is performed, including hysterectomy and/or pelvic floor surgery such as vaginal repair of organ prolapse. The top of the vagina can scar downwards after a hysterectomy or the walls can scar together, affecting its elasticity and significantly shortening the vagina. This can lead to severe pain with intercourse, preventing deeper penetration or preventing intercourse altogether, depending on the severity of the shortening.* 99

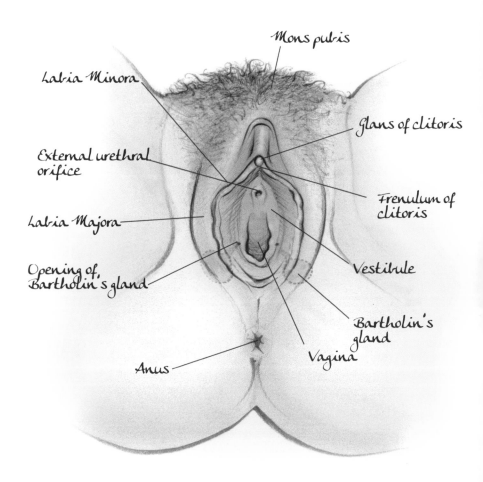

Mons pubis

Labia Minora

Glans of clitoris

External urethral orifice

Frenulum of clitoris

Labia Majora

Vestibule

Opening of, Bartholin's gland

Bartholin's gland

Anus

Vagina

minora, containing the orifice of the urethra - next to the clitoral body, urethral sponge and vagina). Also known as the clitoral bulbs, the vestibular bulbs are part of a collection of erectile tissue, which fills with blood during sexual response, which then becomes trapped within the clitoris causing the clitoris to become erect. When the bulbs become erect they cuff the opening of the vagina in such a way that the vulva expand outwards. The blood that is trapped inside the bulb is released into the circulatory system by the spasm of orgasms. If no orgasm is reached the blood will leave the bulbs over the next few hours following intimacy.

Vulva – is the name given to the lips of the vagina. The big lips on the outside, usually covered by pubic hair, are known as the labia majora and the lips of the inside that cover the vaginal and urethral openings are known as the labia minora.

Clitoris – is a sexual organ surrounding the vagina like a horseshoe, with "legs" that extend along the vaginal lips to the anus. It is the most sensitive part of the vagina, with over 8,000 sensory nerve endings (more than any other part of the body) and is a woman's erogenous zone. Homologous to the penis, the clitoris has the equivalent capacity to receive the same sexual stimulation. Stimulation of the clitoris creates sexual excitement and a clitoral erection and increased sexual pleasure can lead to clitoral orgasm. It is considered key to a female's sexual pleasure.

The clitoral structures surround and extend along and within the labia, as first determined by Masters and Johnson between 1957 and 1965, and thus they concluded that not all orgasms are of clitoral origin. In their initial studies of 382 women, they concluded that orgasmic response was identical whether stimulation was clitoral or vaginal, proving that some women were indeed capable of multi orgasmic expression. Their books Human Sexual Response and Human Sexual Inadequacy, published in 1966 and 1970 respectively, were best sellers and translated into more than thirty languages.

> " *In their initial studies of 382 women, they concluded that orgasmic response was identical whether stimulation was clitoral or vaginal, proving that some women were indeed capable of multi orgasmic expression.* "

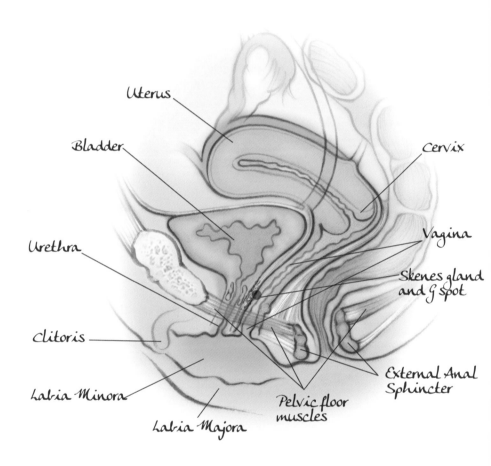

Uterus

Bladder

Cervix

Urethra

Vagina

Skenes gland and G spot

Clitoris

External Anal Sphincter

Labia Minora

Pelvic floor muscles

Labia Majora

Pulled out Clitoris – during arousal and orgasm, the clitoris and the whole genitalia engorge and change colour as the erectile tissue fills with blood and the female experiences vaginal contractions. The female sex cycle has four phases (Masters and Johnson, 1966) and research has shown that a woman can experience a sustained intense orgasm through stimulation of the clitoris and remain in the orgasmic phase for much

In 2005, Urologist Dr Helen O'Connell used MRI technology to note a direct relationship between the 'legs' or 'roots' of the clitoris and the erectile tissue of the clitoral bulbs and corpora (main part of organ), and the distal (location from origin or attachment) urethra and vagina. She notes that the interconnected relationship is the physiological explanation for the conjectured G-Spot and thus the experience of vaginal orgasm, taking into account the internal parts of the clitoris during penetration. "The vaginal wall is, in fact, the clitoris," said Dr O'Connell. "If you lift the skin off the vagina on the side walls, you get the bulbs of the clitoris - triangular, crescental masses of erectile tissue." Her belief is that the clitoris is more than just its glans - the "little hill." Many scientists argue that the G-Spot does not exist, but for those women who have 'heightened' the vaginal canals through pelvic floor exercise - a vaginal orgasm is the most explosive thing you could ever experience!

longer than previous studies had indicated. This is evidenced by the engorged genitalia, colour change and vaginal contractions.

A POINT TO NOTE: IT IS USUALLY HARDER FOR CLITORAL STIMULATION ONCE THE MENOPAUSE BEGINS, BUT NOT IMPOSSIBLE. HOWEVER, VAGINAL ORGASM CAN BE GREATER AND MORE EXPLOSIVE WITH A STRENGTHENED PELVIC FLOOR.

◆ **Urethral sphincter** - the urethral sphincter is a collection of muscles used to control the flow of urine (micturition) from the urinary bladder. The muscles envelop (surround) the urethra to ensure the urethra can be sealed shut when the muscle contracts. There are actually two urethral sphincters in the male human body:

◆ **The Internal Sphincter** muscle of the urethra is located in the bladder's inferior end, and the urethra's proximal (nearest to origin or point of attachment) end at the junction of the urethra with the urinary bladder. The internal sphincter is a continuation of the detrusor (a part of the body that pushes down) muscle and is made up of smooth muscle (as explained earlier); therefore it is under involuntary and autonomic (nervous system) control. This is the primary muscle for stopping the release of urine.

◆ **The External Sphincter** or urethrae, is controlled by the pudendal nerve (somatic nerve within the pelvic region associated with sensation or motion), which acts to constrict the flow of urine through the urethra. It is located at the bladder's distal inferior end in females and inferior to the prostate in males. Unlike the internal sphincter the external sphincter is made up of skeletal muscle, therefore it is under voluntary control of the somatic nervous system. Anatomically, women urinate more than men because our bladders share the same space with the uterus and vagina in the anterior wall. In men, the internal sphincter muscle controls the flow of urine, in women it is the levator ani, the voluntary muscle of the pelvic floor that can be used to control the flow. Because of its involvement in urine flow, any damage to the levator ani can cause a weakness in the sphincter

> " *In Thailand there are women who can inhale cigarettes through their vaginal canal or "spit" ping pong balls and darts!* "

In Thailand there are women who can inhale cigarettes through their vaginal canal and then blow out smoke rings, or "spit" ping pong and darts! Extreme as this may seem, it is the best example I can give you for just how strong the contractions can become once you have trained your pelvic floor muscles and is another reason many men run to Thailand in the hope to have a 'gripping' experience! Inhalation is merely elevation of the pelvic floor and the smoke rings are a gradual co-ordinated descent of the floor, whereas "spitting" demonstrates the power behind a concentrated push/descent of the pelvic floor. The world's strongest vagina belongs to a Russian lady who can elevate 14kg with her pelvic floor - awesome (even if it is a tad disturbing!) Women like this not only have amazing pelvic floor strength and taut vaginas, but they also have contoured lower abdominals and aesthetically pleasing and functional bottoms, and usually nicely contoured legs because the muscles of the bottom help to keep our inner thighs activated, meaning no knock knees and feet without fallen arches! They are almost perfect examples of confidently continent and sexually satisfied females.

5

mechanism (commonly happens during childbirth) and this can lead to stress incontinence. This is another reason why understanding the anatomy of this area and the role of pelvic floor exercises, are crucial to optimal wellbeing.

The Pelvic Floor – sometimes referred to as the pelvic platform, is similar in shape to a hammock or funnel. This 'hammock' is made up of interwoven muscles, ligaments, tendons and connective tissue. It is suspended between the pubic bone at the front, the two sitting bones at each side, and the coccyx at the back, and is about the size of an open hand. Its anatomical name is the perineum.

The pelvic floor acts as a supporting platform to prevent the internal organs and the contents of the abdominal cavity from falling out. It provides openings for the anus and urethra and acts to hold in or release waste, solid or fluid, through these passages. The vagina runs through the middle of it.

The pelvic floor and respiratory diaphragm are physically connected to each other and function more effectively when they work in unison. They are designed to move up and down together whether in contraction or relaxation and this is the reason why correct breathing is crucial to optimal control and function of the pelvic floor.

The fascial system (connective tissue surrounding muscles, blood vessels and nerves binding them) provides a network of functional / sensory feedback, through the nervous system, linking the musculoskeletal system to the core. This synergistic activity should happen voluntarily, without thought or effort. If this is not the case, then the Pelvic Core Nervous System (PCNS) must be trained.

There is a valuable connection between the levator ani and hip (obturator internus) via the arcuate tendon. These are also connected to the abductors and gluteus medialis, which provides an equal and opposite balanced reaction to the hip. All of these interconnections produce a chain reaction activation of the pelvic floor muscles when hip rotation movement is added to core training exercise.

Many women can present with a "tight vagina" when having an internal examination or during intimacy, yet cannot hold their bladder the moment they start any impact work. This is what is known as a "traumatised or overactive pelvic floor." It can either be a result of misprogramming – just squeezing alone, without elevation and keeping the pelvic floor in a constant state of induced tension (which can be detrimental to the pelvic floor in the long term), without the necessary load (impact). Or for many women it is where they subconsciously store all their past issues, disappointments, heartaches and trauma (including sexual abuse such as rape which is forced invasion without consent on the most precious part of a woman's body). Many women have been taught to just 'squeeze' after childbirth, in exercise classes and to stop urine flow, and whilst this may seem like the right thing for the pelvic floor, the action of constant increased tension without the 'right load' does not prepare the 'floor' for a true load, for example during impact exercise and thus it cannot respond and support accordingly.

Many women in frustration, embarrassment or loss of self-esteem and confidence, about the aesthetics of their pelvic floor and lack of sensation, will opt for a vaginaplasty, an operation with costs which start from approximately £2,950. With more women opting for the quick fix, non-educational route in order to make the

> 66 *Many women can present with a "tight vagina" when having an internal examination or during intimacy, yet cannot hold their bladder the moment they start any impact work.* 99

labia (vaginal lips) look 'prettier' and the vaginal canal smaller in the hope of a better sexual experience, this has become a great 'growth' industry which has increased by over 500% since 2007. The problem with this type of operation is the interruption and removal of nerve endings (for which there are millions) in your labia (vaginal 'lips') and when you 'trim' the labia (lips of your vagina) you 'trim away' the nerve endings, removing sensitivity. You may make a smaller entry, which has been stretched after childbirth (but can be stretched by continuous use of big objects also) but you still do not have the muscular and voluntary response you control from a conditioning programme and furthermore, a subsequent pregnancy and delivery can mean more pain during delivery and another operation for a second repair.

Whilst the labia may have been stretched after multiple childbirths, they do not necessarily remain so open as many of the "before surgery" pictures show on internet sites advertising this type of service. A Pelvic Floor Secrets conditioning programme strengthens, conditions and has a "pulling back" effect, which help to "close and shrink the appearance of the opening and labia" so that it does not have to appear so "unattractive." Ultimately, as mentioned before it is how it feels that leaves the biggest and most lasting impression on your husband and partner and makes you both feel euphoric with each intimate encounter. Your pelvic floor and vaginal canal are not made of a material that can or should be placed in a tailor's hands. Rough cotton can have a serrated or jagged edge and can be handled more roughly than the most delicate piece of silk. Neither have feelings or sensory cells and nerve endings. Our private parts don't like scissors and/or stitches and were not designed to be 'nip tucked' unless it is seriously necessary. It would be wise to really think

> " In the United Kingdom the subject of the pelvic floor is still considered taboo. We are still very prudish when it comes to this topic, whilst we are seen as one of the most promiscuous nations in Europe. "

carefully before going under the knife to 'tailor' what Mother Nature gave you as a gift. You may just live to regret it!

In the United Kingdom the subject of the pelvic floor is still considered taboo. We are still very prudish when it comes to this topic, whilst we are seen as one of the most promiscuous nations in Europe. We will not even discuss the subject in terms of and for the sake of our health and wellbeing. Time and again, when I do any workshops or run a master class, it is not usually the English that will be first to book or consider the program, although statistically they have a higher incidence of pelvic floor dysfunction and organ prolapse. I am told time and again, "I will wait until I need to do it."

This has got to be one of the craziest of statements I have ever heard!

Why would you wait until your body begins to embarrass and let you down before you pay attention?

Our apathy or even ignorance for such an important and vital part of our bodies must change. We must choose to understand our body, instead of keeping the continual expectation that the hospitals and doctors' surgeries will put us back to where we never respected we were in the first place.

I am so excited to be the first to offer such a service in Central London. Simply put, offering women (and men soon) the opportunity to be in control of this most intimate part of their bodies at all times in all activities. Pelvic Floor Secrets is the ultimate tightening, conditioning and rehabilitation program for your pelvic floor. It is the first program of its kind

> " *This has got to be one of the craziest of statements I have ever heard! Why would you wait until your body begins to embarrass and let you down before you pay attention?* "

> 66 *Whether you 'Vajazzle' your 'Vajayjay' or give it a 'Hollywood,' now you can not only look great on the outside but you can feel great on the inside too!* 99

to offer exercise targeted specifically toward optimal pelvic floor and vaginal health, and total wellbeing. It is a sensory program that awakens the pathways to the pelvic floor, maximising communication to improve response, tone, strength and support. The end result is a pelvic floor that is positively responsive to all movement, voluntary or otherwise: supportive, protective and enhancing. It is a win-win for women personally, a win-win for women and their partners, and a win-win for the NHS or private medical insurance.

Whether you 'Vajazzle' your 'Vajayjay' or give it a 'Hollywood,' now you can not only look great on the outside but you can feel great on the inside too!

Pelvic Floor Secrets is not a program motivated to just fix. It is an education and empowerment program coupled with the correct pelvic floor exercise program and supporting vaginal strengthening aids, which will all ensure a significant improvement of the pelvic floor. It allows women to run, jump, sneeze, laugh, cough etcetera with a renewed confidence that they will not or no longer leak. Organ support is maintained and orgasms are intensified. The program is tailored to the individual and offered on a one to one basis so that women do not have to feel less confident amongst their peers.

To be confidently continent and sexually satisfied is not a privilege for the chosen few. It is a luxury to be enjoyed by all women of all ages. The pelvic floor is not limited by age or ability, size or social status, but by the accessibility of relevant education and the right strength and conditioning program that ensures you never experience an embarrassing moment again.

The Cervix

Many women only think about their cervix in terms of smears and cervical cancer and, like the rest of this most precious gateway, it is seriously overlooked. But its relevance and importance to reproductive health, sexual pleasure, support of the organs and overall optimal health should never be dismissed. I believe it is VITAL that we as women truly understand its roles and responsibilities if we are to really believe we desire optimal health.

The role of the cervix is to:

◆ Promote fertility. As we orgasm our cervix descends into the pool of semen within vaginal canal increasing the chance of pregnancy
◆ To allow the flow of our menstruation
◆ Protect the uterus, upper reproductive tract and the developing fetus from pathogens (infections)
◆ Play a role in sexual pleasure by heightening the contractions felt within the vaginal canal, assisting in the constriction of the perineum, anal and vaginal sphincters
◆ Provide support for the bladder (pubocervical fascia)
◆ Provide support for the upper part of the pelvic floor by the cardinal ligaments (supported to the lateral pelvic sidewall) and uterosacral ligaments (run from the sacrum to the cervix).

The cervix is very firm and is the lower part of the uterus. It acts as a stabilizer for the fascia (connective tissue) of the female pelvis. It is known also as the cornerstone of the upper female pelvic floor just as the perineum is the central support for the lower part of the lower pelvic floor. The cervix and perineum are the centre points for stabilisation of the pelvic floor. It is a weakness within either one or both of the cardinal and uterosacral ligaments that causes a prolapse of the upper vaginal, uterine, vault or an enterocele. A cystocele (prolapsed bladder) is caused by a weakness in the pubocervical fascia (connective tissue).

It is important to recognise the role of the cervix in protecting the uterus from infection. The uterus usually lies across the top of the bladder, but stands more 'erect' during arousal and penetration allowing the cervix to dip into the vaginal canal and pool of semen. Thus sexually transmitted infections (STI's), such as Gonorrhoea, Chlamydia, HIV and HPV (human papillomavirus – most common especially between 16 – 18 year olds) which are transmitted with intercourse and ejaculation mean the cervix whilst protecting the uterus becomes the primary site for infection and is the reason why these infections can pose a huge health risk for cervical health.

Whilst no test is foolproof it is for this very reason that the PAP smear is so important. The late Jade Goody admitted to missing one or two of hers and the opportunity therefore to prevent such a detrimental outcome. Since the introduction of the smear test in 1928 the death rate of cervical cancer has been reduced by up to 99% in the US where screening is routinely done. In other countries including the UK, where it is not carried out as routinely or its importance and/or relevance not made common knowledge from school age, the death rate is 74%. With the increase in promiscuity and teenage sex, this information should really be a mandatory part of the school curriculum. The American Congress of Obstetricians and Gynecologists (ACOG) recommend that screening should start from the age of 21. They believe that young women should wait for a couple of years after becoming sexually active before having their first smear. The UK starts it screening program much later and this can be questionable since

66 *The late Jade Goody admitted to missing one or two of hers and the opportunity therefore to prevent such a detrimental outcome.* 99

young girls are engaging in sexual expression at a much earlier age and most young people who contract HPV tend to do so soon after they become sexually active.

A PAP smear does not hurt although it may be a little uncomfortable, but it can be the difference between a healthy or unhealthy outcome. A speculum is inserted into the vagina in order to take sample cells from the surface and canal of the cervix. These cells are then sent away to a lab where they are checked for abnormal cell growth, also known as dysplasia (abnormal changes in the cells on surface of cervix), cervical intraepithelial neoplasia, CIN (pre-malignant transformation and abnormal growth of cells on surface of cervix).

What is important to note is for every 3.5 million women tested, only 13,000 are likely to have true cancer, which if caught early does not have to result in death.

The cervix also plays a role in the support of the bladder via the pubocervical fascia (connective tissue) and whilst many women do report having an improved sex life or no change in orgasmic explosion, without understanding its importance and the vulnerable position the bladder is placed in, they may find themselves suffering from a prolapsed bladder later, if increased strength and conditioning of the pelvic floor does not become a mandatory part of their exercise regime.

5

When Pain Becomes the Biggest Motivator

PAIN has always been a great motivator for fixing or seeking a solution to a problem or condition. We are a nation of reactionaries. We react to pain, based on the severity of the symptoms. We ask the questions after the fact. Much like the police after a road traffic accident when trying to establish cause and fault, we hope we can improve prevention and save another from suffering, instead of acquiring or using the knowledge beforehand.

The pelvic floor is an amazing platform. It brings an immense amount of pleasure for those women who have educated themselves on its rewards, and who can enjoy its benefits intimately, with the confidence that its primary role of support and protection is not compromised by default. These women are not motivated by pain, but rather reward.

However, for as many as 75% of women, this is not the case. Many women are offended by the word "vagina", the correct anatomical name for this part of the body. It is like a swear word to them and I find this amazing. Comfortable to 'disguise' it by any other name, women then do not seek to find out its weaknesses. Just because pelvic floor muscles are hidden doesn't mean women can ignore them. It is not a topic of conversation that is entertained or entered into. We know it is the gateway for sex and for elimination, and it is the gateway that brings forth life, yet most childbirth stories focus on the pain.

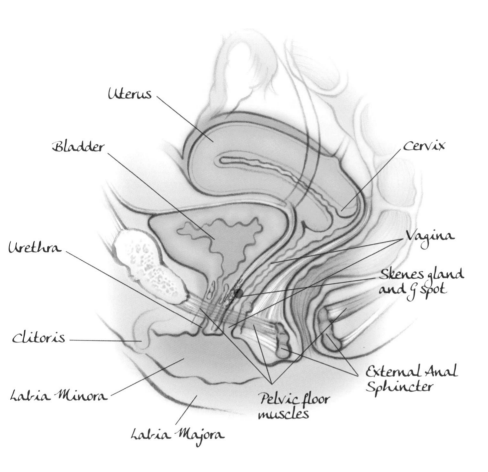

Chapter Six

Uterus

Bladder

Cervix

Urethra

Vagina

Skenes gland and G spot

Clitoris

External Anal Sphincter

Labia Minora

Pelvic floor muscles

Labia Majora

We are a nation and world that is driven by sexual images, videos, innuendos and fantasies. We want to be seen as sexy and are motivated towards that end, but we do not understand the true function of the vitally important pelvic platform that runs right through the vagina and "holds up" our internal organs and because of that it can be a very painful revelation for an increasing number of women.

> *We are a nation and world that is driven by sexual images, videos, innuendos and fantasies. We want to be seen as sexy and are motivated towards that end, but we do not understand the true function of the vitally important pelvic platform that runs right through the vagina and "holds up" our internal organs,...*

Dysfunction and the Pelvic Floor

There are many dysfunctions that can befall the pelvic floor, but two of the most debilitating are incontinence and/or prolapsed pelvic organs.

Pelvic organ prolapse is increasing at an alarming rate amongst a much younger population of women, and consultant gynaecologists are struggling to understand the reasons why. If the consultants are struggling then what hope does the average woman have?

In order to answer that question you have to have the knowledge of the role of the pelvic floor and the things that can adversely impact it and bring about such an outcome.

Interestingly, it is Hispanic and Asian women who tend to suffer the most from prolapsed pelvic organs when compared with Caucasian women (who are more likely to have a hysterectomy); whilst black women are the least likely to suffer. There are numerous sources of information available on this matter (Springelink and the American Urogynecologic Society to name a couple), but whilst no one is conclusively sure why this is, they do believe it may be a lack of access to appropriate information. And whilst statistically this may be correct, I am increasingly encountering Caucasian women in their early to mid-thirties who are suffering from organ prolapse after their first or second child.

The primary role of the pelvic floor is to support or "hold up" the upper part of the vagina, bladder, bowel and rectum which sit directly above it. The gravitational pull we have on our pelvic floor, caused by everyday activities such as standing and walking around is often overlooked. The fact that the pelvic floor sits just above the vagina and all of the organs above sit on it, means that in the standing position the pelvic floor is required to provide far more support and the gravitational pull down is increased. Any weakness in the pelvic structure results in a downward movement or the bladder, uterus or even the rectum falling towards the vaginal canal. Any of these can cause a continual loss of urine with activity, problems with bowel movement or even an uncomfortable bulge within the vaginal canal or vaginal opening.

Pelvic floor problems are virtually non-existent amongst mammals as walking around on all fours means they do not experience a continued gravitational pull as we do. The pelvic floor is also responsible for the support of all our internal viscera; intestines and abdominal structure. That is a lot to support, particularly with gravity adding to that load. Based on this information alone, we women should begin to have a fair idea about the enormity of the continued load we place on this pelvic floor of ours. This pelvic floor was built to last for primal man and the way he lived. The way we live today however, is very different from the simple life of hunter, gatherer and thus our pelvic floor is put under exceeding pressures, leading us to require a maintenance program in exactly the same way you would service a car in order to optimise performance and longevity. However, our pelvic floors need this maintenance on a regular basis.

> *Pelvic floor problems are virtually non-existent amongst mammals as walking around on all fours means they do not experience a continued gravitational pull as we do.*

The actions that can affect the pelvic floor are:

- ◆ Coughing
- ◆ Laughing
- ◆ Sneezing
- ◆ Walking
- ◆ Running
- ◆ Jumping
- ◆ Pushing
- ◆ Pulling
- ◆ Lifting
- ◆ Twisting
- ◆ Turning
- ◆ Bending

All of these are natural movements that we make regularly without thought or regard. We may have to run for a bus, we might jump when we are cheering for our kids at sports day or for our favourite team. We squat, lunge, reach up to get something off the shelf, etcetera, and all of these movements come under push, pull or lift. Every time we make any of these movements there is a downward force through the abdominal viscera that is buffered by the pelvic floor. Our pelvic floor used to be able to cope with these movements, in the era before everybody started running for fun, or to lose weight quickly, or increased their high-impact exercise.

> " Every time you strike the pavement it is up to seven times your body weight that goes through your joints and pelvic floor. "

Our pelvic floor was designed to support these organs and maintain them in their rightful place, whilst carrying out all these activities and going through childbirth. But we have added to that load in our drive to look good. Aesthetics has become our motivator without any regard for the increased stress we put our bodies or more specifically our pelvic floor through to achieve it. Every time you strike the pavement it is up to seven times your body weight that goes through your joints and pelvic floor. Do the maths on an average nine stone female running at a pace of 215 steps per minute, for 30 minutes at a time:

$$9 \times 14 = 126\text{lbs} \times 7 = 882 \times 215 = 189{,}630 \times 30$$
$$= 5{,}688{,}900 \text{ lbs of stress!}$$

6

That is the kind of force you put your body through for a single road run and all that pounding is impacting on your hammock-like sling which is constantly working to make sure everything remains in place as you run. Increased impact work is a major contributory factor to a weakened pelvic floor, struggling to maintain the organs in place.

Understanding the role and responsibility of the pelvic floor and then ensuring it is continually strengthened and conditioned will allow you to do impact work with confidence.

It should be the initial training program before all exercise if its role of support is to be maintained with confidence.

Ten years ago when the 'core' became the buzzword, we were being told to 'set our core', without the relevant education for the reason why or the responsibility of this muscle. For the most part, we were not really aware of what it was and how we should activate it correctly. In September 2005 I published the book, *Can a Vagina Really Buy a Mercedes? What can your pelvic floor do for you?*

66 *Understanding the role and responsibility of the pelvic floor and then ensuring it is continually strengthened and conditioned will allow you to do impact work with confidence.* 99

That book looked directly at the link between the lower abdominals and pelvic floor – our core, and the exercises that could help it. The women that followed the advice are amongst those who have continued testimonial success.

Ten years on and we are now talking 'pelvic floor core', recognising in this growing industry of incontinence and prolapse, that the pelvic floor is an integral part of the core and must be managed as such. But, whilst it is an integral part, it must be identified and exercised appropriately as the foundation exercise before an impact or load program is fully introduced, and this is where the gyms are not delivering. It is not because they cannot, but it is because they do not offer short-term classes that are beneficial for life (not seen as economically viable), and secondly it is because there is still a stigma attached to the pelvic floor, which says, "Unless you are suffering, you do not need to worry." Hello! This is rubbish!!! And it is precisely why so many women are suffering, because they did not worry about their pelvic floor in the first place.

But once the body has reached the point where problems with the pelvic floor are evident, people tend to look for the quick fix. As a society we want everything instantly. We are generally not prepared to work towards so many things and I believe this is the reason so many marriages are failing. Everything in life requires work and maintenance; our friendships, relationships, jobs, dreams and aspirations. None of these things just happen overnight. It is a constant battle to maintain a good relationship and to be able to work through the continual conflict that comes up daily, weekly or at another interval, but it is the love and respect, or bigger picture that allows us to endure.

This is the same for the pelvic floor, our overall bodyweight and image. They all require a level of dedication commitment and above all the right education to ensure you can optimise your wellbeing and outcomes. When the police look over the scene of a road traffic accident, it is in the hope to improve prevention. It is the same for the pelvic floor! *"If you know and you do, you will emerge a winner, improving prevention."*

When it comes to the pelvic floor, the statement, 'knowledge is power,' really does apply. Ladies, if we really desire great aesthetics we need to start with what is inside. There is no point looking hot, when the mind is full of darkness, anger, sadness etcetera, because your eyes will reveal your true emotions. Your skin, nails, eyes, hair and posture will reveal how well you eat and drink, and your health reveals your lifestyle habits, both dietary and environmentally. The effectiveness of your exercise program is obvious in your posture above all else, and your pelvic floor success is obvious to the trained professional, in the shape of your bottom, lower abdominals and posture (especially visible in legs). So whether you are aware of it or not, you do advertise your knowledge of self.

Look at that final statement and think about what you advertise and sell on a daily basis. Is it confidence, subconscious or otherwise as well as either a distinct understanding/ respect for your health and wellbeing OR a lack of understanding/disregard for it?

With the education and confidence that you function well, you are able to go about your daily tasks with less stress. To be noticed and/or elevated within the work place requires not only the aptitude for the job but an outward display of your confidence in your abilities, and this is always easier when you naturally outwardly

> 66 *When it comes to the pelvic floor, the statement, 'knowledge is power,' really does apply. Ladies, if we really desire great aesthetics we need to start with what is inside.* 99

Here is part of a poem I wrote in 2007:

An ode to your body

*They say your body is your advert – and you
know this must be true – each day it tells a
story, each day the story's new!
You advertise your life, your health and who and where
you're at, and without a care for what it says your
advert could be flat!*

.

*The health of all your organs, your cells and all within
can be told, as your story unfolds through your hair,
your nails, body shape and skin!
A healthy spine, strong bones and joints
should be important too.
They play their part in posture and
the perception of you!*

.

*Your teeth - your visual story, say most about who you
are and when they're good your story's great and
peoples view are fair by far!
Dad always said, "Your hair's your beauty"
so investment here is great - it shapes the face God
gave you, and plays its part in fate!*

.

A welcoming expression and great posture too can
signify a confidence, the right attitude and self-esteem
that will always elevate you!

So before you pay no attention, step back and stop
and think, 'cos what you say and how you look
should really be in sync!
Your body is your advert - make sure you advertise well
- like any other advert
you only reap from what you sell!

display that. If confidence were available on a shop shelf, trust me,
it would be continuously out of stock. Confidence inspires, motivates,
rewards and keeps you pushing forward. Pain or embarrassment on the
other hand stagnates and can stop you in your tracks. *Pelvic Floor Secrets*
is not meant to be a sex book, or a book that reprimands, but rather a
guide to pelvic floor practices that reward your diligence, attention to
detail and obedience and discipline when it comes to looking after such a
precious bit of kit. Let's face it, we are motivated by rewards and bribes,
and a good friend of mine who works as a top barrister once said, "There
is nothing wrong in offering a 'bribe' if it gets you the right outcome!"
I am of course talking legal bribes, just like the ones we offer to our
children every day in exchange for their cooperation.

We live in a nation where some 85 - 90% of the population do not
exercise or eat the healthiest diet. Looking after ourselves is something
we have chosen not to take responsibility for.

> **We live in a nation where some 85 - 90% of the population do not exercise or eat the healthiest diet. Looking after ourselves is something we have chosen not to take responsibility for.**

We say, "It's my body, I can do what I want," or, "It's my body, you cannot dictate to me what I can or cannot do." Yet, when our body begins to fail us, we believe that because we pay into the NHS we have the right to hold an expectation that they will fix us. Good or great health has almost developed a class system of its own.

Think about the amount you pay for your national insurance contributions and then think about your health. Is this really all the value you have placed on your health? There are two things we cannot buy: health and time. We are told to use our time wisely; this means good life choices, not just good material choices. It means good health choices and good conscious choices that impact not just you, but others, and for the better.

In the Bible, Joshua 1:8, God tells Joshua to, "Meditate on the word day and night and not let it depart from your lips and then you will have good success and be prosperous." I love this verse, even though, like a fool I do not follow it always. It tells us that if we apply God's word we cannot lose in ANY area of our lives, and that prosperity comes from obedience. Think then of your health; if you acquire, understand and apply all of the principles of healthy living 80% of the time, you still have 1/5th of your life for letting your hair down and indulgence. Proverbs 3:2, "For length of days and years of life and peace they will be added to you" – this is God's promise to Christians who trust in the Lord with all their heart. If you trust in your health and do not forget what you are being taught and follow the health ratio, then this too can be your portion in life. Remember, it is not sensible to expect long days, long life and good health, with bad dietary and lifestyle habits.

Pelvic floor health is affected by both dietary and lifestyle choice. Its full function is dependent not just on the right strength and conditioning program, but also on the accessibility of the right nutrition to keep the muscles healthy.

You do not need to tie yourself into some marathon training sessions followed by a diet of lettuce leaves. In fact we must move away from the myth that good food is rabbit food. It is far from it, and apart from feeding the cells within the pelvic region it is important to feed the cells within the brain, the heart and other internal organs as well as our limbs. Why not let the body have optimal nutrition at least 80% of the time? Why not be responsible for your own health and not hand it over to a doctor who knows very little about your journey, dreams or aspirations? Don't ask the doctor to "fix you" - you fix you! Invest in your health and the education you need to keep it, in the same way you would invest in your home.

You get a mortgage, life insurance, just in case, and then you tie yourself to your job to allow you to buy all of the trimmings and accessories. Trim and accessorise your health by learning to breathe diaphragmatically, letting oxygen flow freely around the body and eliminating stress blockages and ill health. Understand your pelvic floor and the impact of every movement you make upon it. Understand the principles of movement and movement patterns, and get off machines bolted to the floor that cannot possibly transfer to daily routines and go back to basics. Value sleep as this is the time that the body repairs, regenerates, replenishes and refreshes.

> *In fact we must move away from the myth that good food is rabbit food. It is far from it, and apart from feeding the cells within the pelvic region it is important to feed the cells within the brain, the heart and other internal organs as well as our limbs.*

> **Be in control of the content of your food. Get back into the kitchen and cook – the only additives in your food should be the ones you add!**

And last but not least,

Be in control of the content of your food. Get back into the kitchen and cook – the only additives in your food should be the ones you add!

It is impossible for a doctor to be able to go through all these variables with a fine-tooth comb, second guessing which or what component may be the main culprit, and if you are not listening to your body, how do you really expect a doctor to know where to begin, other than a generic pill bottle that has been proven to make somebody "be seen to feel better."

My Pelvic Floor, something you cannot see
Can either reward or debilitate me!
I can choose to ignore it and not value its role
Then under the knife I may just have to go
Extra protection I need when I laugh
And, 'the feeling' in intimacy... a memory that's past
Or I can choose to acknowledge, condition and enjoy
"Gripping" and "lifting" and jumping for joy
A little attention, a few minutes a day and
I can confidently..., 'continently...' be on my way.

6

Prolapsed Organs

The number of women who have or are suffering from a degree of uterine or bladder prolapse after their first child is increasing rapidly, and these are women who have access to the best medical and physical services, private health clubs and private medical health.

For these women and many others, to suffer dysfunction after childbirth is not only embarrassing but it is debilitating. Many top gynaecologists, doctors and health care professionals believe that this one condition alone (especially urge incontinence) is more detrimental to a woman's quality of life than many other serious diseases such as diabetes and even some cancers.

> **Many top gynaecologists, doctors and health care professionals believe that this one condition alone (especially urge incontinence) is more detrimental to a woman's quality of life than many other serious diseases such as diabetes.**

This is because many women no longer feel confident to leave the house for fear of embarrassing themselves in public.

Up until now you will have had to suffer from some degree of pelvic organ prolapse before you could gain access to the limited services that are available, and even once you gain access, the information/education and relevant strength and conditioning programs can leave women feeling disheartened, with a sense of hopelessness about their full recovery. All of this has a negative impact on a woman's confidence that then affects her relationships both at work and at home, and over the long term can be a contributory factor to marriage and relationship breakdown. Thankfully, with Pelvic Floor Secrets, you can begin to enjoy the changes that can become noticeable within as little as six weeks.

Prolapsed organs are painful both physically and psychologically, and it is this pain that is the motivator to seek assistance. Even then, many women wait until the degree of prolapse has a seriously adverse effect on their lovemaking before they go to see their GP for a referral to a gynaecologist. This is crazy!

Hidden from view, not a thought or regard – the pelvic floor
Your internal bodyguard!
Put under pressure all day and all night,
To avoid embarrassment the sphincters must stay shut tight.

.

The organs that sit on it can dislodge from their home and then
into the vaginal canal they may roam,
The pain and discomfort then motivates you
To seek a solution to
Repair and resume

.

Sensorial in nature
The last pathway to wake
Needs constant conditioning for confidence sake

.

The foundation of your trunk is your pelvic floor
To support and protect as if a trap door
Understand it well and value its role
'Confidently Continent' be it your goal.

Phillipa

Phillipa came to my Swiss ball class in London, in April 2010.
She approached me at the end of a class after I included one
of the pelvic floor exercises from my first book and she then
emailed me her experience during labour. She had pushed for
two and a half hours during her first labour and 20 minutes
during her second. The result was a grade 2 uterine prolapse in
September 2009, which meant the uterus had descended into
her vagina.

She had been working with a specialist physiotherapist over
the previous eight months doing basic kegel exercises and
had the strength of the contractions measured by electronic
pulse, which hovered at around 12 microvaults - less than
what is considered normal or average. A contraction strength
greater than 15 is considered to be normal/average. Yet after
five sessions in my "group" exercise class, the strength of the
contractions measured had increased to 15 and then up to the
dizzy heights of 23 (her words), demonstrating two things:

◆ A significant improvement of the strength and
condition of her pelvic floor
◆ That these muscles can be improved in a relatively
short period of time, enough to avoid surgery

Phillipa was signed off from the physiotherapist in June 2010
and her prolapse was now registered as a grade 1. She says,
"The workout is great fun and has made me feel physically
fit in the rest of my body too." It has given her back her

femininity. As for her kegel's 'clicking' she says: "Bring it on!" My favourite statement came when she invited me into her home and her husband said, "Thank you for giving me my wife back!"

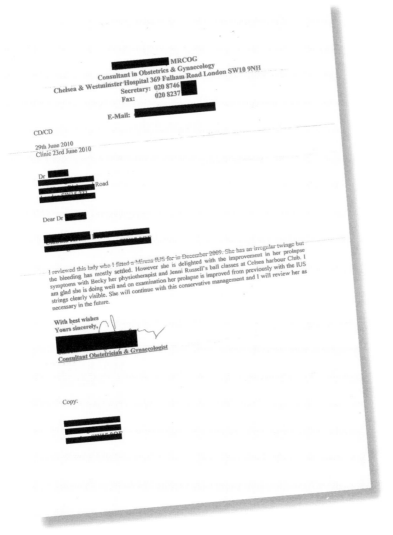

■■■■ MRCOG
Consultant in Obstetrics & Gynaecology
Chelsea & Westminster Hospital 369 Fulham Road London SW10 9NH
Secretary: 020 8746 ■■■
Fax: 020 8237 ■■■■
E-Mail: ■■■■■■■

CD/CD

29th June 2010
Clinic 23rd June 2010

Dr ■■■■
■■■■■■■ Road
■■■■■■■■

Dear Dr ■■■■

■■■■■■■■■■■■■

I reviewed this lady who I fitted a Mirena IUS for in December 2009. She has an irregular twinge but the bleeding has mostly settled. However she is delighted with the improvement in her prolapse symptoms with Becky her physiotherapist and Jenni Russell's ball classes at Celsea harbour Club. I am glad she is doing well and on examination her prolapse is improved from previously with the IUS strings clearly visible. She will continue with this conservative management and I will review her as necessary in the future.

With best wishes
Yours sincerely,

■■■■■■■
Consultant Obstetrician & Gynaecologist

Copy:
■■■■■■■
■■■■■■■

Rebecca

Rebecca came to me in the middle of 2010 when I began a Swiss Ball Pelvic Floor Clinic in SW18, also known as nappy valley. I set up this new clinic thanks to Phillipa, who wanted to spread the empowerment in her community. It was a lovely intimate class with six women in their early thirties. The majority of these ladies had given birth to one child and had then suffered pelvic organ prolapse. The beauty of intimate classes is that women are confident enough to open up and share their pelvic floor dysfunctions, as they said, "We are all here for the same reason," even if our conditions are different.

Rebecca had a common bond with Alexis in that they had both suffered a cystocele, a bladder prolapse, with Alexis attending after having had an operation known as bladder bulking (use of Botox to assist in ensuring the urethral sphincter can maintain continence). Rebecca was scheduled to have bladder taping within three weeks of the six week course. Alexis explained that the operation had only been a success for around three weeks. This was because, as she lay on the operating table having the anaesthetic she was told to ensure she did not lift anything heavy for six weeks post op. This is absolutely crazy. How can a new mum with a little baby not pick her child up? I always tell my clients that your child is just that first and a weight second, so if the average baby weighs around 6-7 ½ lbs at birth, then three months on they may weigh as much as 18-22lbs (just shy of one stone) or even more - this weight alone in the gym for many women is a challenge.

Alexis said the operation was wonderful; having suffered from incontinence for many years, after the procedure she was ecstatic that she could hold her urine. But she had a child to look after and a husband that worked, and like many mums, she had a limited support network, so she was forced to attend to most of her baby's needs herself, and this included picking him up. The operation was undone within three weeks, which was why she was at my class exploring another avenue. She warned Rebecca not to consider this operation as an option. Rebecca chose to have the TVT procedure (Transvaginal Taping), bladder taping. The TVT sling procedure can be performed as an outpatient procedure with minimal pain and a short period of recovery (although this was not Rebecca's initial experience). Whilst lifting is restricted for 6-8 weeks and no sex is allowed for 4 weeks minimum, many women can then resume what is considered a 'normal life.' The TVT sling acts as the hammock, false pelvic floor, to support the urethra, as the original pelvic floor should whenever you cough, sneeze or exercise etcetera. However, nothing artificial can ever be as good as the sensory systems that already exist in the body. Understanding these systems is key to optimal pelvic floor health and wellbeing, and is a crucial part of really knowing and understanding your body.

Rebecca had her operation the following week and initially everything that could go wrong did. When she tried to ask questions of her consultant before the operation she found herself with either inadequate answers or none at all, as the allotted time did not allow for this. And just like Alexis, as

7

she was about to have her operation, she was told, "Do not lift anything heavier than a kettle." What Rebecca found hard was the realisation that she was the only young mother having the procedure (she said that all the other women present on that day were elderly) and after the operation she had a few complications that kept her in hospital for two days, whilst everyone else seemed to go home that afternoon. Her consultant flippantly said to her, "Don't worry, 1 in 15 suffer a complication!" That is a relatively high number.

I am so pleased to report that Rebecca had a positive outcome in the end. Whilst she says she wishes she had met me earlier, or that physiotherapists should be recommending a service such as mine, she is able to maintain continence.

A POINT TO NOTE: IT IS IMPORTANT TO NOTE THAT A NORMAL LIFE, AS DESCRIBED ABOVE, MUST INCLUDE A CONDITIONING PROGRAM FOR THE PELVIC FLOOR. WHILST THE TVT SLING HAS REPORTEDLY BEEN SUCCESSFUL IN 90% OF CASES, THIS SUCCESS RATE HAS A SHELF LIFE OF APPROXIMATELY THREE TO FIVE YEARS. THIS IS BECAUSE WOMEN ARE BEING BADLY INFORMED OR ARE NOT DOING THE RELEVANT CONDITIONING PROGRAM TO MAINTAIN PELVIC FLOOR STRENGTH. THE SLING IS LIKE A PROP, OR THE ORIGINAL LIGAMENTS, WHICH NEED THE ASSISTANCE OF THE CONDITIONED PELVIC FLOOR IN ORDER TO ENSURE THAT IT WILL NOT LET YOU DOWN IN THE FUTURE.

Ladies, don't wait until you experience pain or dysfunction before being motivated or forced to take action. Many of my clients tell me the sense of hopelessness comes when the surgery date is set, even before physiotherapy begins. At the Vitality Show in Kensington Olympia in March 2011, women admitted to me that they would "wait until the pelvic floor began to let them down BEFORE they would worry about it!" This is absurd! Doctors prescribe and set surgery dates. Physiotherapists work on the point of pain with the limited time allocated. CHEK trained healthcare professionals consider the whole body as a kinetic chain and understand that wherever pain is, it usually originates from somewhere else, and it a small part of a bigger issue.

Pelvic Floor Secrets is not just this book, it is a series of workshops and a clinic, offering a range of sensory programs that ensure the correct recruitment of the pelvic floor and transverse abdominal muscles before strength training can begin, whether you are pre or postnatal, just wanting to awaken your pathways, preparing for your wedding night or dealing with special conditions. It includes the best vaginal strengthening products, organic 'raw' supplements by PureXP as well as a Metabolic Typing nutrition and lifestyle plan so that the outcome is working towards optimal health and wellbeing of the whole body. The results can be experienced in as little as six weeks; rewarding you with improved physical function, sexual pleasure and aesthetics.

Surgery should never be the first recourse for patients to experience or the GP to offer as a means of 'correcting' a dysfunctional pelvic floor.

They should start with a corrective exercise program. Surgery is a quick or deemed immediate fix, without any education of how or why your body found itself responding as it did and any 'cutting' of sensory receptors just makes the area weaker over time as the sensory system has been 'interrupted'.

> " *Surgery should **never** be the first recourse for patients to experience or the GP to offer as a means of 'correcting' a dysfunctional pelvic floor.* "

Whilst many women report short-term improvements, they can experience a not so pleasant outcome in the long run. More awareness is needed of the roles and responsibility of the pelvic floor as well as its rewards, especially as people are motivated by reward rather than work. Kegel exercises, named after Dr Kegel, are usually only mentioned as a passing statement to the patient that has just given birth, as if they are the only ones who can be affected by a dysfunctional floor. Alternatively they may find they are just given a sheet of paper without a full explanation of what, why and how, and this is a major problem.

Kegel exercises don't seem to be understood by healthcare professionals. The concept of isometric vs isotonic is consistently dismissed. Many healthcare professionals, up until recently, argued that the pelvic floor could not be engaged from 'front to back,' and still see it as a chore themselves. Many of these same professionals do not have good health practices as individuals, so the easiest answer is surgery.

There are various pelvic organ prolapses that can happen, and understanding what, why and how can help you to avoid any of these. By maximising the efficiency and health of your pelvic floor you can prevent having to memorise the symptoms or experience any of the causes:

Uterine prolapse

A prolapsed uterus literally means a displacement of the womb, sometimes referred to as a pelvic floor hernia – a downward displacement of the uterus from the upper vagina, causes it to lower or 'fall into' the vaginal canal. In more severe cases, a complete displacement can mean that the cervix is visible through the opening of the vagina itself and as mentioned in chapter five, can make it vulnerable to infection. The cervix supported by the cardinal and uterosacral ligaments provide the support for the uterus and fallopian tubes. A weakness in either or both of these ligaments is what allows the prolapse to occur. As the cervix is integral to the upper

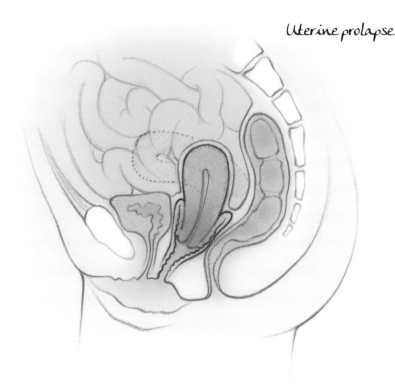

Uterine prolapse

pelvic floor, a laxity in this support system is a weakness in the pelvic floor and thus will increase the chances of organ prolapse.

Around 20% of women have a 'retroverted uterus' also known as a 'tipped uterus' which literally means that the uterus tips towards the back (more upright as it does during intercourse, so the cervix can descend into the vaginal canal during orgasm and ejaculation) and this can increase the risk of prolapse. A 'tipped uterus' is aligned with the vaginal canal and may or can be subjected to a "piston-like effect" that occurs from the intra-abdominal pressure when the abdominal muscles are used – as in excessive crunches – which can push the uterus down into the vagina.

Many women, myself included, tend to find that this condition is reversed after childbirth.

A prolapsed uterus is usually more prevalent in Caucasian women, as well as women who have had multiple vaginal births or given birth to large babies. The uterus does not always prolapse immediately after childbirth (which usually happens with white women after their second or third child) and may appear many years later (which tends to happen in African or Caribbean women in my client experience). If no attention has been paid to the pelvic floor muscles, during these pregnancies, deliveries and life thereafter, the muscles are understandably considerably weaker and thus become ineffective in their role of support.

There are a number of symptoms of uterine prolapse, the first of which is the feeling or sensation that something is coming down through the vagina. There can also be a sense of fullness within the bladder or rectum. In addition, there may be a "dragging" discomfort of the lower abdomen, low backache, heavy menses and mild vaginal discharge. Women may also experience an increase in frequency of urination, but tend to find it difficult to totally empty their bladder, which can then become infected causing burning when using the toilet. As if this is not bad enough, women can also become constipated or find it difficult to pass stool, and lastly, dependent on the degree of prolapse, women can find that normal sexual intercourse becomes difficult and pregnancy no longer possible.

A POINT TO NOTE: IT IS IMPORTANT TO UNDERSTAND THAT THE POSITION OF THE BLADDER AND RECTUM WHEN SEATED ON A TOILET SEAT ARE NEVER OPTIMISED, AS THEIR ANATOMICAL POSITION WITHIN THE TRUNK REALLY REQUIRES US TO BE IN A DEEP SQUAT POSITION ALLOWING THE ORGANS TO 'FACE NORTH' AND THUS EMPTY COMPLETELY. PLACING YOUR FEET ON A STOOL AND KEEPING THE TRUNK ELONGATED, IMPROVING POSTURE, HELPS, BUT OPTIMALLY

PLACING THE THIGHS AGAINST THE TUMMY IS BEST FOR COMPLETE EVACUATION (SEE SECTION ON THE TOILET SQUAT ON PAGE 27).

Many factors can contribute to uterine prolapse including:

◆ Continuous distension of the intestines because of either gas or excess food matter. Either of these will cause a constant downward pressure on the womb
◆ Chronic constipation which causes pressure in the back passage because the colon is too full
◆ Tight clothing (especially corsets)
◆ Constant stooping – note this is different from deep squatting
◆ Weak or weakened condition of the lower abdominals, through lack of exercise or correct exercise prescription (see Visceroptosis on page 24)
◆ Overall body condition
◆ Prolonged labour and/or interference in delivery (forceps etcetera)
◆ Lack of adequate rest and poor diet choices in postnatal phase
◆ Repeated delivery (especially back to back)
◆ Manual work which can increase the weight on the womb
◆ Tumour of the uterus
◆ Traction of the uterus and/or surgical injuries
◆ Menopausal atrophy

Incidentally, it is easier to prevent prolapse of the uterus than to cure it after its occurrence. One of the most fundamental measures to prevent this is to understand the role and function of the pelvic floor and to pay attention to the maintenance of it, via simple easy to execute exercises for all women. Good antenatal care during pregnancy is much easier with the understanding or education of the pelvic floor, which puts you in a more empowered position. And whether you like it or not, there is such a thing as good vaginal health, impacted by our diets, so you really do need to understand not just the importance but the impact of including relevant foods for optimal nutrition. This will help to normalise weight, and help to avoid becoming constipated which would otherwise put unnecessary pressure on the perineum and pelvic musculature.

Cystocele

A cystocele is a fallen bladder, which usually occurs when the wall between the bladder and vagina – the pubocervical fascia (connective tissue) - is torn, common during delivery in childbirth. It is this fascia that separates the bladder and urethra from the vagina. As long as it remains intact it assists in preventing the bladder from bulging down into the vaginal canal. All prolapsed organs are 'graded' in terms of their severity or how far they descend toward the opening of the vagina and 'the outside world.' A grade 1 is considered mild and can be maintained with a 'comprehensive' pelvic floor program, as can grade 2. Sometimes a grade 1 or mild cystocele may only be noticed by a physician or nurse, during a routine examination, and cause no pain or discomfort to the patient. A grade 2 or 3 (mild or severe) prolapse will present with symptoms that become increasingly 'annoying' as the patient experiences problems emptying their bladder. They may also experience a feeling of pressure in the pelvis and vagina, especially when bearing down. This can lead to repeated bladder infections, urinary incontinence and even pain during sexual intercourse. A grade 3 prolapsed organ is within the vaginal canal itself and can still be maintained with a comprehenive program and be regarded on examination, dependent on discipline and conditioning to a grade 1-2 avoiding surgery. A grade 4 is when the organ is actually visible or totally outside of the vagina and 'hanging'. Once a patient has left the prolapse to get to this stage an operation is usually the only or best solution.

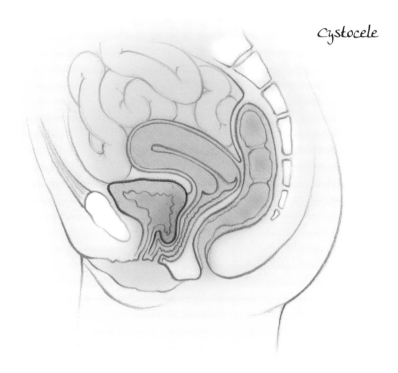

Cystocele

I have worked with many women who have a grade 3 prolapse and have been able to reverse this to a grade 2 or grade 1-2, avoiding surgery, acquiring the relevant education and homecare to protect themselves and preserve their femininity.

As with uterine prolapse, it is easier to prevent prolapse of the bladder than to cure it after its occurrence.

Again, one of the most fundamental measures to prevent this is to understand the role and function of the pelvic floor and to pay attention to the maintenance of it, via simple, easy to execute exercises for all women (yes I am repeating myself, but it is necessary). Again, with cystoceles, good antenatal care during pregnancy, as mentioned above, is much easier when coupled with a confident understanding or education of the pelvic floor, which puts you in a more empowered position.

A POINT TO NOTE: AN ANTERIOR WALL REPAIR OF THE BLADDER PERFORMED BY MOST SURGEONS CUTS AWAY THE PART OF THE BLADDER WALL THAT PROVIDES SUPPORT FOR THE UTERUS (PUBOCERVICAL FASCIA) AND USUALLY LEADS TO A UTERINE PROLAPSE! IT IS VERY IMPORTANT FOR YOU TO ESTABLISH EXACTLY WHAT PROCEDURE THEY INTEND TO PERFORM AND TO VERBALISE THAT YOU DO NOT WANT ONE PROBLEM SOLVED TO CREATE ANOTHER MORE DEBILITATING ONE FOR WHICH THE USUAL ANSWER IS A HYSTERECTOMY. A TOTAL LOSS OF YOUR FEMININITY!

Rectocele

A rectocele happens if the thin wall of fibrous tissue (fascia) that separates the rectum from the vagina is weakened. This weakening allows the front wall of the rectum to bulge into the back of the vaginal canal.

The bowel is the lower part of the digestive system: from the stomach to the back passage. The small intestine is what is known as the lesser bowel, where the food you eat is digested and the nutrients absorbed. The large bowel, also known as the large intestine, is where the water from the digested food is held and this helps to form stool.

The main factor that can affect the fascia, by placing unusual or increased pressure on it, is childbirth. With pregnancy, the ligaments, tendons and fascia that hold and support the vagina can become weakened and then childbirth/delivery can weaken them further, causing the rectum to 'drop into' the vagina, leading to constipation, and piles. Heavy lifting and obesity also place undue pressure on the fascia and the greater the load, without correct conditioning and support, the more opportunity there is for dysfunction.

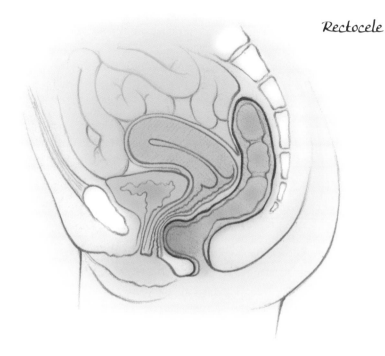

Rectocele

Rectoceles vary in size/degrees, and a small rectocele may have no symptoms or signs. However, a large rectocele may cause a bulging of the tissue through the vaginal opening, which may be very uncomfortable. It is rarely painful physically. A larger rectocele can make bowel movements very difficult and the sufferer may need to use their fingers to press against the bulge in the vagina to help push the stool out during the movement. In many cases there is usually a sensation as if the bowel is not fully emptied or rectal pressure or fullness.

Rectoceles can be a very embarrassing prolapse for women and can stop them from being intimate with their husbands or partners. A feeling of vaginal 'looseness' (laxity) is also experienced with this type of prolapse.

Left unmanaged many women go on to experience another prolapse, either:

- ◆ Cystocele – bladder
- ◆ Enterocele – small intestine
- ◆ Uterine – uterus

Another reason for ensuring good pelvic floor practices, as mentioned above, is they are easier to prevent than to cure.

Enterocele

An enterocele is also known as a vaginal hernia. It occurs as a result of the small intestine (small bowel) descending into the lower pelvic cavity and then pushing on the top part of the vagina, creating a bulge. They are most common in women who have had a hysterectomy. The two are very closely linked as part of the small intestine lies just behind the uterus in the space known as the pouch of Douglas.

Once again, childbirth can have a negative affect because of its impact on the pelvic floor and so too can age. It is crucial to understand the role and responsibility of the pelvic floor if you are to avoid one of the many prolapsed organs. The pelvic floor supports the bladder, uterus, colon and small intestine, and any weakening in its strength and condition can lead to one or more of the dysfunctions mentioned above.

Symptoms include:

- ◆ A feeling of pelvic fullness, pressure and/or pain
- ◆ A pulling sensation in the pelvis that decreases when lying down
- ◆ Lower back pain also easing when lying down
- ◆ A soft bulge of tissue in the vagina

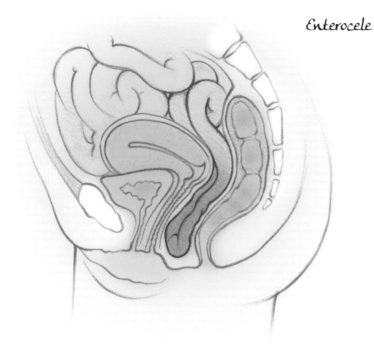

Enterocele

◆ Vaginal discomfort
◆ Painful intercourse (dyspareunia)

Like other organ prolapses, chronic coughing, constant heavy lifting (causing intra-abdominal pressure), constipation, obesity and multiple childbirths can all have long-term detrimental effects on the pelvic floor. The issue of age should be of concern to everyone, as with age there comes the possibility of weakened connective tissues. These tissues support the organs in their anatomical position and they can become overstretched leading to the organs being dislodged (prolapsed).

Pain and Embarrassment

I WAS talking with a colleague at work and he suggested that I focus primarily on the incontinence market, as it is such a big one! There are approximately six million reported cases of incontinence in this country, but it is believed that the actual figure could be as high as 50% of the population. Incontinence is the most underreported condition, and one that an increasing number of men are beginning to suffer with.

The one overriding factor though is that incontinence is *not painful*; it is *embarrassing*! Women are great at hiding embarrassing ailments and continence pads allow you to maintain your condition discreetly. So confident are the manufacturers of these, that they have amazing adverts on TV showing women getting caught in an embarrassing situation with a lovely looking man, but he has no idea of her true embarrassment; frightening!

> " *Whoever told women that incontinence is a part of the aging process, lied! Incontinence is a result of the forgotten de-conditioned pelvic floor.* "

Whoever told women that incontinence is a part of the aging process, lied! Incontinence is a result of the forgotten de-conditioned pelvic floor.

The hidden sling, just above the pubic bone, the foundation of the torso. It is not held up by muscles alone but rather ligaments that do not do well if they are not given the extra support that the conditioned pelvic floor muscles provide.

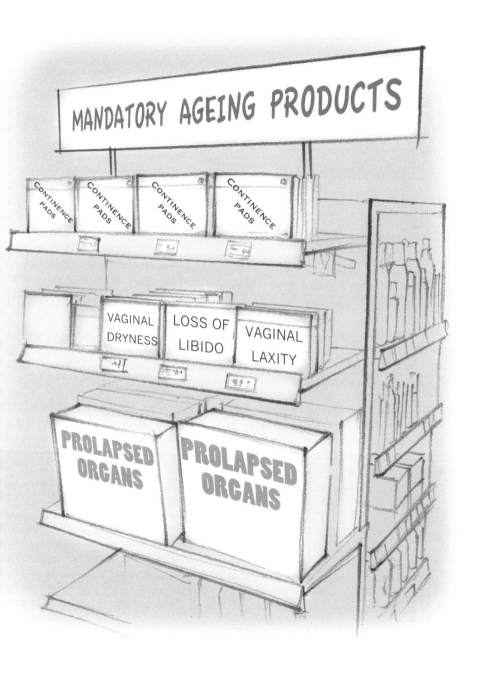

Chapter Eight

Continuing to mask a problem does not make it go away; physically and/or mentally the condition must be faced in order to manage and/or eliminate it. Come on ladies, the vagina is self-cleaning, which is why we are not supposed to continually douche or use fragrant soaps, for fear of upsetting the pH balance, or washing away the bacterium that protects the canal from infection. If the body were designed in such a way, why would it want to let us down like this unless something

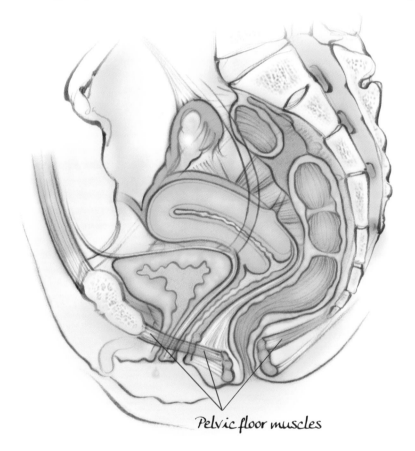

Pelvic floor muscles

has gone wrong? Personally, I hate embarrassment. I try to avoid it at all costs, and if I do experience it, I seek to ensure that I do not find myself in that situation again. Unfortunately, this is not the case with continence pads, which keep you in the same state: ignorance. Incontinence on a large scale can impact all daily activity.

Planning a simple social evening for an incontinent lady is often focussed around the proximity to the toilet. They will always wear dark, loose clothing. The latest pastels will not be a part of their wardrobe. Detrimentally, they stop drinking water in the hope that they will not need to visit the toilet, risking dehydration of the organs and the pelvic floor, which is vital to optimal health. Intimately, they become withdrawn, and at work they worry about being seen to be taking too many toilet breaks, or worrying about relaxing too much during social conversation. Ignorance, laziness and a lack of accessibility to the relevant information can stop women from changing these outcomes.

8

A great example was given by top gynaecologist Mr Mark Slack on the BBC Radio 4 show *Woman's Hour*, where he pointed out that a patient suffering with urge incontinence may run for a train, just catch it and as they drop into their seat the full contents of their bladder empties. They may only want to go two stops, but the embarrassment will root them in their seat until the carriage is empty, which could well be the end of the line.

Urine and your bladder

Our kidneys continually make urine, and a trickle of that urine constantly passes to the bladder, via the ureters (tubes from the kidneys to the bladder). The amount of urine we make varies, dependent upon our consumption of food and drink, and how much we sweat. The bladder is a muscular storehouse for urine, which expands like a balloon as it fills. The urethra is the outlet for urine (also the same outlet for orgasmic fluid) that is normally kept closed by the muscles within the pelvic floor that envelop around the urethral sphincter. Sensory signals from the brain, to the bladder and the pelvic floor, let us know when the bladder is getting full and thus we are able to go to the toilet voluntarily. As you urinate, your bladder contracts and squeezes, whilst the pelvic floor muscles and urethra relax.

The two most common types of incontinence are:
◆ Stress incontinence
◆ Urge incontinence

Stress Incontinence

The most common form of urinary incontinence is stress incontinence, affecting approximately 1 in 100 adults in the UK. Ladies, the sad news is that 1 in 5 of us will begin to suffer this type of incontinence from the age of forty... (and this is more commonly seen in obese women).

Associated with physical stress such as exercise, coughing, sneezing, jumping, running, twisting, turning etcetera, it can be exacerbated after childbirth or with age and/ or lack of 'correct exercise prescription'. The pelvic floor muscles and the urethra, if functioning optimally, can

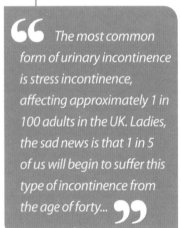

> " The most common form of urinary incontinence is stress incontinence, affecting approximately 1 in 100 adults in the UK. Ladies, the sad news is that 1 in 5 of us will begin to suffer this type of incontinence from the age of forty... "

In April 2011, Whoopi Goldberg and Kris Jenner (the mum from the *Keeping up with the Kardashians* TV show) fronted a campaign for the Poise brand that quoted 'Famous Women in History' (including Cleopatra, Mona Lisa and Lady Liberty) who achieved great things, but also suffered from what they eloquently termed "Light Bladder Leaking" (LBL). The aim of the campaign was to let us know that even the most famous women can suffer the same affliction and yet still achieve greatness.

"Like millions of women, I have my own experiences with LBL, but I've never let it keep me from living life to the fullest," said Kris. "Inspired by the impact that last year's 'Great Women in History' series had on women with LBL, I've teamed up with the Poise brand to help women understand that LBL is common and manageable so it shouldn't stop them from doing great things and being the incredible and accomplished women they are."

Whilst this is true, it is equally true that to become enlightened and empowered could mean you need never become an LBL woman, but rather a CC one - "Confidently Continent" - amounting to great things and enjoying life to the fullest without the embarrassment of adult nappies masking as pads!

8

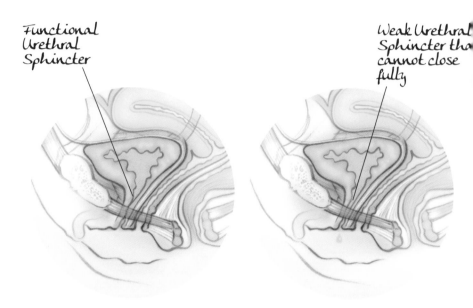

Functional Urethral Sphincter

Weak Urethral Sphincter tha cannot close fully

withstand this type of sudden pressure and avoid any leakage, but the opposite is true if they are weakened. It is important to understand that the body is indeed a kinetic chain and that nothing happens without it impacting neighbouring muscles, which have a knock on effect.

The pressure within the abdominal wall, as explained earlier, is known as intra-abdominal pressure, which can cause a downward force with every movement if there is a dis-coordination between the upper and lower abdominal muscle regions (look at the pictures right: normal or optimal breathing - as the respiratory diaphragm moves down, the lower and upper abdominals move in and the pelvic floor is elevated up, however, if there is a dis-coordination and the lower abdominal move out as the upper abdominals move in then the buffer, lower abdominals cannot stop the 'load' falling onto the pelvic floor and thus it moves down as it become abnormally loaded). If the organs of the abdominal

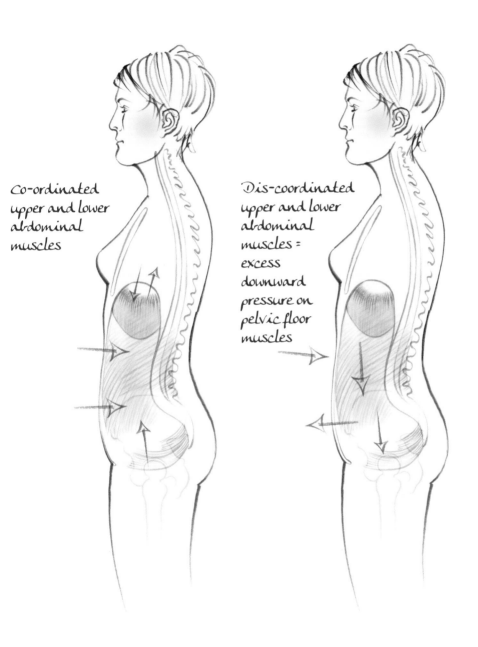

Co-ordinated upper and lower abdominal muscles

Dis-coordinated upper and lower abdominal muscles = excess downward pressure on pelvic floor muscles

8

structure continue to bear down on our pelvic floor, aided by gravity, then without any regard for the maintenance of the floor, we leave ourselves open to a continued downward pressure of the organs that sit on it, which over time can prolapse into the vaginal canal.

Urinary stress incontinence is more embarrassing than it is annoying or painful. It is usually believed to be as a result of childbirth, but this is not always the primary cause. Heavy lifting, weak lower abdominal, buttocks and external rotator (hip) muscles, as well as poor posture, all have a massive impact on the strength and condition of the pelvic floor, directly affecting the urethral sphincter which can also cause this condition. In many cases stress incontinence can also occur as a result of the urethral sphincter becoming hypermobile. Hypermobile muscles are muscles with extra movement. This is not good, as a urethra with too much movement inhibits its ability to close (do its job) properly on a continuum. This condition can occur as a result of weakened pelvic floor muscles that:

◆ Become overstretched as a result of de-conditioning
◆ Allow the bladder to sag downward within the abdomen. The sagging bladder then pulls on the internal sphincter (muscle around the bladder neck) which is attached to the urethra

A POINT TO NOTE: SOME MEDICAL PROFESSIONALS DO REFER TO INCONTINENCE AS THE FIRST STAGE OF PELVIC ORGAN PROLAPSE. URETHRAL HYPERMOBILITY CAN BE CATEGORISED BY EITHER TYPE 1 OR TYPE 2 HYPERMOBILITY.

◆ In Type 1 hypermobility the bladder neck and urethra can remain completely closed
◆ In Type 2 hypermobility the angle of the bladder neck shifts. In many cases a cystocele results.

Our urogential and reproductive area is made up of smooth muscles: 70% slow twitch (tonic) and 30% fast twitch (phasic) fibres. Phasic muscle contracts and relaxes rapidly, whereas tonic muscle contraction is slow and sustained. Tonic muscle fibres can maintain force over prolonged periods with little energy utilisation and are the reason why we are able to 'make it' to the bathroom. Tonic muscles allow us to hold urine without feeling under any pressure in terms of energy output. Our everyday activities require our pelvic floor to be able to maintain good endurance, which is why we have a dominance of slow twitch fibres. Thus the importance of using the "right acute exercise variables when conditioning the stabiliser systems, which is rarely ever done by both rehabilitation and/or exercise professionals" - Paul Chek (Lancashire interview June 2012). However, sudden bursts of activity or increases in load require the muscle to contract quickly to allow for the increase in intra-abdominal pressure, this is where the fast twitch fibres are required.

Women who suffer from stress incontinence are usually able to 'hold on' and make it to the toilet, but find that when they sneeze, laugh, cough, jump, etcetera, they lose a little urine. Their phasic or fast twitch muscles are not quite contracting on time to stop this loss. This is because of the sudden surge in intra-abdominal pressure, which forces the internal organs downwards onto the pelvic floor (see exercises on page 192). Whilst this may be embarrassing for women who suffer stress incontinence, it is those who suffer urge incontinence who find their lives debilitated by it.

Intrinsic Sphincter Deficiency (ISD)

Intrinsic sphincter deficiency is another major cause of stress incontinence in women. It occurs when the muscles within the bladder neck are either damaged or weakened and this can cause one of two things:

- The bladder neck opens during filling
- The pressure around the urethra is too low to allow the internal sphincter to close fully. This usually occurs in women after previous surgery

What are the Treatment Options for Stress Incontinence?

The great news is that for 6 out of 10 cases of urinary stress incontinence, significant improvement or even elimination of this condition can be seen with the correct pelvic floor exercise program. Although many of us shy away from exercise, pelvic floor exercise significantly impacts our confidence, self-esteem, sexuality and our relationships. No other exercise program has such a major effect on our confidence the way the pelvic floor does.

Surgery

Surgery may be advised if the problem persists and pelvic floor exercises have not worked well, which in many cases is usually due to a lack of discipline or diligence to commit to the correct and full execution of the exercise program.

> " Surgery should always be the last port of call, as it is not an education on how the muscle works, but rather a short-term solution to an issue that will undoubtedly re-occur. "

Various surgical operations are used to treat stress incontinence. These tend to only be used when the pelvic floor muscle exercises have not helped (or are deemed to be unsuccessful as mentioned above). The operations aim to tighten or support the muscles and structures below the bladder. In some women, medication and pelvic floor exercises may be advised instead of surgery. This is usually in women who do not want to have surgery or who have health problems that may mean that surgery is not suitable.

A POINT TO NOTE: ALL OF THE MUSCLES IN OUR BODIES ARE FED BY SENSORY RECEPTORS AND IT IS THESE RECEPTORS THAT ARE INTERRUPTED DURING ANY OPERATION, LEAVING LESS SENSORY RECEPTORS TO HELP THE ALREADY WEAKENED MUSCLES RESPOND.

Surgery should always be the last port of call, as it is not an education on how the muscle works, but rather a short-term solution to an issue that will undoubtedly re-occur.

Can Stress Incontinence be prevented?
If you make regular pelvic floor and related exercise (see exercise section in chapter 13) an integral part of your daily routine, not just during pregnancy and after you have a baby, then stress incontinence is less likely to develop, even following childbirth and in later life.

Urge Incontinence
Urge incontinence, also known as an overactive bladder, is when a woman is 'unable to hold on' and make it to the toilet. Their tonic or slow twitch fibres are not able to do their job optimally. Unlike stress incontinence where they tend to lose only a little urine, urge incontinence can be a total emptying of the bladder, which is why it can become so debilitating. Women with urge incontinence usually need to urinate many times throughout the day, up to as many as 12 to 14 times. This can have a massive impact on their relationships at work, and at home (intimately), which can lead to relationship breakdown and ultimately lead to a total isolation of the patient. The fear of embarrassment, whether whilst out shopping, going out with friends or on an overnight stay with friends or family, can make a patient imprison herself at home. Women are even frightened to run for the bus or train for fear of sitting down and voiding, as mentioned above.

8

> For a young girl who is still at school, incontinence can have the most devastating impact on their education and social skills. And for many adults, the Council's lack of understanding as to the enormity of the problem with regards to less and less public toilets can exacerbate the problem. It is funny that many of us have no regard for public toilets. We treat them with little or no respect, and the cleanliness of these toilets reflects this.

Intimately, an overactive bladder can mean that many women urinate at orgasm, making them very uncomfortable about having sex and thus having an adverse effect on their relationship. Whilst there is medication available that can cure the incontinence, it is not yet known whether this medication is also the cause of associated vaginal dryness, so much so that lubrication becomes a problem leading to painful penetrative sex. We really can be put through the mill!

The limited service that is available to correct urge incontinence, leaves many women who are suffering with it with a sense of hopelessness about the outcome.

> " The limited service that is available to correct urge incontinence, leaves many women who are suffering with it with a sense of hopelessness about the outcome. "

A poor response to the rehabilitation program and/or a lack of sensitivity from the physiotherapist can destroy any confidence of a positive solution for the patient. Pelvic floor exercises must be effectively explained, and the healthcare professional explaining them must ensure the patient understands the sensory program first. The sensory program is the program that dictates the success of any pelvic floor rehabilitation program. You have to be in tune with your pelvic floor if you are to expect it to work toward optimal health and improved sexual function. *Pelvic Floor Secrets* is the only program that offers a comprehensive sensory program of good practices.

'Is there a right time to have incontinence surgery?' The answer can be yes, but only if the symptoms have become too dramatic for the sensory system to work without assistance.

A POINT TO NOTE: THE QUESTION THAT MANY SURGEONS ARE ASKED AFTER THIS OPERATION IS, "WHY DID I WAIT FOR SO LONG, OR SUFFER SO MUCH?" IF YOUR BLADDER BEGINS TO LIMIT YOUR ACTIVITIES, EVEN WHEN YOU HAVE STOPPED PLAYING SPORTS, HIKING, JUMPING ON THE TRAMPOLINE WITH THE CHILDREN, OR CARRYING OUT MANY OTHER EVERYDAY ACTIVITIES. IF YOU ARE FORCED TO WEAR A MINI-PAD OR ARE EXPERIENCING LEAKAGE EVEN ONCE YOU HAVE FINISHED HAVING CHILDREN, THEN BEFORE YOU CONSIDER SURGERY, CONSIDER GETTING TO KNOW YOUR BODY INTIMATELY FIRST. YOU MAY JUST SURPRISE YOURSELF. A LITTLE SENSORY TRAINING OR RE-TRAINING AND YOU MAY JUST FIND YOURSELF DRY ONCE AGAIN, IN AS LITTLE AS SIX WEEKS; WITH LITTLE COST AND NO OPERATION, JUST AN INVESTMENT IN TIME WHILST YOU GET TO KNOW YOURSELF.

Fix it or Mask it
Continence pads are a great way to maintain your condition discreetly. But discretion is not the best choice neither is it a solution. It is amazing that we train toddlers out of nappies at the age of two years, yet we indulge in adult "nappy pads". Because the necessary education and information is not as freely available as an immediate discreet solution is, women are not encouraged to work towards eliminating the problem but rather to mask it. This is backed up with the belief that it is a part of a woman's cycle of life, as sold by the marketing companies and those who continue to profit from our ignorance. We may be

masking it well, but the NHS with its recent cutbacks has targeted the incontinent woman. How much more embarrassing and debilitating must it be for a woman in old age to have to bring three soiled pads into an incontinence clinic, so that they can be measured to ensure their level of soaked urine qualifies them to free continence care? As if your dignity is not challenged enough. Let this be an incentive again to ensure you do not find yourself in this horrific position.

According to the manufacturers of a well-known continence brand, the statistics for incontinence show that globally it affects around 5-7% of the population and this figure grows by approximately 4% per annum. Europe accounts for 40% of the market and just fewer than 30% of the market can be found in North America.

The increasing aging population is one reason given, but my experience in the clinic and from my many masterclasses, is an emerging group of younger, more active women who have found themselves having to look for more discreet ways to manage their condition. For a certain company supplying continence pads, they have been able to become the global market leader, with up to 25% of sales for incontinence care in over 100 countries. They actually have just under half of the business within Europe, a 41% share. Astounding!

Institutional care and home care accounts for 62% of this company's global incontinence market. For companies like this, the main focus is on supplying high-quality products combined with qualified advisory services that simplify handling procedures and reduce costs for care providers. The retail market is now the fastest growing segment for continence pads, accounting for 38% of the global market.

The companies supplying these products provide support through information, advertisements and the development of products that are increasingly discreet, easy to use and effective. But they do not provide an education that is either remedial or preventative.

Incontinence is big business, and whilst there is no global program that educates women to empower themselves, for example through an exercise maintenance program, or a media platform where this subject will be discussed more openly, then companies like this will continue to dominate the market. And with their amazing advertising program, which reaches the widest audience, they will continue to maintain the belief that this is the only or best solution.

8

Menopause and your Pelvic Floor

PELVIC floor health is seldom thought about when we are young and vibrant. We cannot see it, and for many women, especially those who have never experienced vaginal births, it is believed that there is no need for concern. Yet this vitally important gateway that links our inner and outer worlds, the most powerful part of a woman's body can be the most debilitating and embarrassing issue that a woman ever has to deal with, especially as she approaches her mature years and the body begins its transition via the menopause.

We tend to associate all ailments of the pelvic floor with age, and the menopause is the first visible sign that our bodies give us to let us know we are indeed, going through the change that brings us toward maturity or aging. But it is how we manage menopause that will dictate how we enjoy the 'second' part of our lives.

> **The symptoms associated with the menopause, such as hot flushes, vaginal dryness and vaginal laxity to name a few, can make life very hard (and even depressing) without having the added worry of prolapsed organs or incontinence**

The symptoms associated with the menopause, such as hot flushes, vaginal dryness and vaginal laxity to name a few, can make life very hard (and even depressing) without having the added worry of prolapsed organs or incontinence (which by the way is considered by many healthcare professionals as the first stage of organ prolapse), which may be as a result of the de-conditioned pelvic floor as well as diet and lifestyle choice.

Chapter Nine

It is funny because throughout our younger years we see periods as the bane of our life, an interruption to our lovemaking, an inconvenience to our training program, or just coming at the wrong time. Yet a period signals our real womanhood, a sign of fertility (for most women). Yet when we go through this transitional stage and the periods begin to become irregular and eventually drop off, we suddenly realise that our biological clock is telling us that natural reproduction in our lives is coming to an end and that can be very hard on some women, especially those who may have chosen to put their career before starting a family, only to have this transition come earlier in their life than anticipated.

This chapter is very dear to me as I write from first-hand experience. At 49 years of age, still full of energy and ideas and in a relatively new relationship, I do not consider myself ready for the other side of the hill as far as my body is concerned, but as I am going through this transitional period known as perimenopause, I have had to begin to make adjustments to lifestyle; eating, drinking, sleep and even exercise habits to make this as smooth as possible. My pelvic floor health has always been vital to me. It impacts my sexuality and my relationship, as well as my overall confidence, aesthetics and wellbeing.

Pelvic floor health is fundamental to any relationship, even the relationship you have with yourself. As women we have many symptoms to contend with at this time; hot flushes, drier skin, thinning hair, mood swings etcetera, not to mention the debilitating issues that come with vaginal atrophy, laxity or dryness:

Vaginal atrophy

Vaginal atrophy, also known as atrophic vaginitis, is the thinning and inflammation of the vaginal walls, due to a decline in estrogen. This estrogen deficiency can also affect the density (thickness) of the internal urethral sphincter (muscles at the bladder neck), thinning it so that it becomes difficult to close fully and thus contribute towards incontinence. Vaginal atrophy normally occurs for most women during or after the menopause, and the bladder capacity tends to decrease. However, this can also happen to some women during breastfeeding or any other time where the levels of estrogen production decline. Healthy genital function is closely interlinked with a healthy urinary system.

Vaginal laxity

Vaginal laxity, also known as a loose vagina, is when the connective tissues supporting the vagina become loose as a result of:

◆ Too much sexual intercourse (without a comprehensive strength and conditioning program to counterbalance the continuing relaxation of the vagina as it expands to accept the penis)
◆ Childbirth
◆ Old age

A loose vagina is usually experienced or associated with women going through the menopause (although in my 15+ years as a pelvic floor expert, an increasing number of women in their early twenties are experiencing this condition) or those who have had a big or multiple birth(s). Promiscuity does have its negative side and too much sex especially from an early age, without recognising the long-term implications for vaginal health can leave women with a sense of "openness" within their vagina – unable to feel their partners or achieve sexual satisfaction. Most men prefer a woman's vagina to be small and tight, allowing for a better sexual experience (and ladies, men do discuss us our "downstairs" with their mates and even work colleagues). There is no such thing as a standard vagina size (although the average size of the vaginal canal is mentioned earlier) but a guide to vaginal laxity is:

◆ You find it hard to 'grip' your index finger with your vagina.
◆ Your vagina is unable to close completely even when you are not aroused.
◆ You find it harder to orgasm than before.
◆ You find it hard to satisfy your partner.
◆ It is possible to insert more than two fingers inside your vagina.
◆ You need to insert larger objects in order to be stimulated.

Vaginal dryness

Vaginal dryness is a very debilitating and sometimes painful expression of the menopause. As we enter this phase of our life, our levels of estrogen begin to decrease, along with our progesterone levels (although many women can experience this without the menopause symptoms). As we are no longer producing eggs and have little or no periods, our bodies no longer require elevated levels of estrogen from a reproduction viewpoint. Any interruption in hormonal balance can make our lives suddenly very challenging. Unfortunately, for total health, a reduction in this hormone can have a negative impact not only on the moisture within the vaginal canal but also on its laxity (tightness). The skin and support tissues of the lips (vulva) and vagina become thinner as a result of the drop in hormone levels and this is the cause for the

9

dryness. The weakening of the pelvic floor then begins and the end result could be incontinence and/or pelvic organ prolapse. Vaginal health therefore has never been more important.

A POINT TO NOTE: PELVIC FLOOR MUSCLES THAT ARE TONED AND CONDITIONED INCREASE THE BLOOD FLOW WITHIN THE VAGINAL CANAL WHICH IN TURN INCREASES THE FLUIDS. ORGANIC GHEE IS A VERY GOOD SEX LUBRICANT AS WELL AS VERY SUPPORTIVE OF THE 2ND CHAKRA ENERGIES - PAUL CHEK (LANCASHIRE INTERVIEW JUNE 2012).

Janie Turner is a former nurse and midwife and author of two Thermomix recipe books. Passionate about creating "A Nation That Eats Well and Cooks With Joy!", she says: "Lots of women who are menopausal experience dryness of the vagina and discomfort or even pain with intercourse. Often they don't know how to talk about this with their partner, so they just endure the pain... the sad thing is that without realising it, they often portray to their partners a subconscious reluctance to have intercourse, so their partner doesn't push it, and the frequency of intercourse diminishes. An easy way to increase lubrication and enjoyment is with cold-pressed organic coconut oil – a teaspoon or two rubbed on the labia and just inside the entrance of the vagina helps immensely and nourishes the area beautifully with all the goodness of coconut oil."

I thank Janie that she has kindly given a recipe from her book "Fast and Easy Indian Cooking" for making your own homemade ghee in your Thermomix, which you can find at the back of the book.

By the grace of God, vaginal atrophy and laxity are not symptoms I have suffered with. Although I have paid attention to this area for years, the menopause and the change in my hormone levels mean I also have to pay particular attention to my dietary intake (including water) in order to ensure that vaginal dryness is not my portion. My suffering, aside from the summers, involves slightly drier skin and hair loss on the left side along the hairline above my ear – not a place that can be readily covered with ease. I am telling you this because the many symptoms of menopause bring about their own esteem issues.

In my poem *'An Ode to your Body'*, I include a line about hair: "Dad always said your hair's your beauty so investment here is great. It shapes the face God gave you and plays its part in fate," and I truly believe that. In the summer of 2011, there was an article in a newspaper about maturing women and hair length, which was subsequently discussed on a breakfast talk show. Whatever the case, your hair, hair quality, style and length, complete everything you put on. Your make-up does not complete your face, your hair does; so when it begins to break or fall out, it is hard to control your levels of stress over it, which incidentally can make the situation worse. Luckily for us, wigs and hair pieces can look very natural indeed and thus allow us to mask the cause of our stress, but this is not the case with the pelvic floor and its impact on our intimacy. This is especially true since many women are also starting new relationships at this time and therefore have to have the confidence for the intimacy they are about to experience with someone new; someone who is yet to know, appreciate and accept their changing body.

> " To ignore vaginal health is to set yourself up for one of the many dysfunctions that are associated with it, therefore vaginal and pelvic floor health are crucial, especially at a time like this "

To ignore vaginal health is to set yourself up for one of the many dysfunctions that are associated with it, therefore vaginal and pelvic floor health are crucial, especially at a time like this.

A maintenance program that includes pelvic floor exercises as a central theme, will assist in helping to keep the pelvic floor strong and stable and also help to keep the area lubricated and plump. Increased water intake is also crucial as water is the hydrator of all the systems of the body including the pelvic floor and vaginal canal. There are also natural progesterone creams and organic herbal supplements that will assist in rebalancing the hormones so that the pelvic floor can remain healthy for life.

The menopause does not have to signal a downturn in any woman's life. As we head towards our retiring years, these should be the most fruitful, rewarding us for the investments we have made during the course of our working life, and that investment should be both physical (in terms of exercise and lifestyle choice) and financial. Understanding your body and how it works, and being able to make the necessary adjustments to keep it working the way you want it to work, is the most empowering position you could ever find yourself in.

The reason I pay attention to this vitally important gateway, the most precious part of my body, is because I fully understand (from client experience and their testimonials) how it could stop me in my tracks. It could adversely affect my confidence and thus my ability to focus on the really important issues and it could halt my relationship. I have not had a period for six months now (since March 2011) and I am not sure how I feel about it. At 49 I am not really looking to start motherhood again, but it is quite debilitating to know that this is no longer my choice. The hair loss and dry skin, not my choice; the personal summers, not my choice. But aside from experiencing a natural birth again, none of these are my destiny either, simply because adjustments to lifestyle and eating and drinking habits can have a major positive effect at halting or reversing these symptoms.

Serenity progesterone cream is interesting. I ordered some two months ago and at first the summers became wildfires – whoosh! But they are beginning to disappear. I can get through a day or two without one and that is significant. I am now on Peruvian Maca and Cocoa powder, which is great for improving testosterone levels and balancing hormones, crucial for a girl like me whose hormones have taken their own field trip without permission. The pure cocoa, which is a major antioxidant, along with the Maca has caused my libido, which is already high, to go through the roof, but my hormones will begin to regulate and that is youthful in itself. For me, this time of my life, is the only time I will drink champagne in celebration of a period, a sign of fertility and youthfulness. Still a 'complete' woman!

> " To lose your libido and not try to get it back can be detrimental not just to your relationship but more importantly, how you move forward as a person. "

9

To lose your libido and not try to get it back can be detrimental not just to your relationship but more importantly, how you move forward as a person.

To ignore vaginal health is to set one's self up for the many dysfunctions that are associated with it, all of which have a long-term adverse effect on self-esteem. I thank God every day for my hubby. I have someone I can journey into maturing age with. We have different goals and aspirations for later life, but for now we are neither old nor feeling old. I do not look old and I do not act old. I am not ready to write myself off and neither should you be. I am looking forward to hitting 50 (Nov 2012), by God's grace. I have looked after my health and I have looked outside of myself to see how I can help to improve the lives of others (this book being a part of that journey) and I love my heavenly Father with all my heart.

These are the supplements, which are a part of my Pelvic Floor Secrets program:

◆ Hydratante from Pure-XP, Superfood, Wheatgrass and Glisodin (Pure-XP).

Hydratante flies off the shelf in Harrods – a complex supplement that includes high-grade fish oils and hyaluronic acid, which helps to maintain the plumpness of smooth muscle, of which the vaginal canal is one, and it is also important for skin health.

Wheatgrass helps to alkalise the system, which is important to help balance our lifestyles and offset environments where disease likes to live.

Glisodin stimulates the body's own hormones to help fight free radical damage.

These supplements can help improve vaginal health but it is vital that I also eat well, according to my metabolic type. I used to joke that any man I meet would say, "You spent how much on food?" My extravagance is not just material. I value the quality of the food and supplements I put into my system and you should too. Do not let studies tell you that organic is a con. If they are offering an organic product it will not contain as many additives, and/or have fewer pesticides used in its production. Growth hormones in poultry manifest in the wings, so you should avoid eating them. Animals that are allowed to forage naturally have better muscle density and it is the muscle that we eat.

Unbleached sea salt is hard to find in the shops, so order it from the Internet. Not only is it better for optimal health, it makes the food taste divine. And lastly, do not forget to use fresh herbs. Again they give food a totally different flavour and the aroma is so inviting. Food shopping should never be cheap, it should be appropriate to optimising your health and wellbeing, all of which assist in longevity and the ability to fully enjoy retirement; slowing becoming a reward for the chosen few. If you shop wisely you can spend £45 - £60 on three meats and get at least six days of dinners, so in the long run that works out at a couple of pounds per head, which is cheaper overall.

Other vitamins and minerals that can be very good for the optimal health of the vaginal canal and for breast health are:

Zinc: A necessary element in the healthy reproduction of cells, the process of repair and growth and an important immunity booster. A deficiency of zinc along with estrogen can have a negative impact on sexuality. Zinc assists in the function of vitamin A and the production of histamine. Histamine levels are needed to help women achieve orgasm. Tissues are also aided by the presence of zinc in the body, helping to prevent many of the body's organs from deterioration and dysfunction.

Magnesium: Every organ in the body, especially the heart, muscles, and kidneys, needs the mineral magnesium. It also contributes to the make-up and strength of our teeth and bones.

Most importantly, magnesium activates enzymes, contributes to the production of energy and helps to regulate calcium levels as well as copper, zinc, potassium, vitamin D, and other important nutrients in the body.

> " Every organ in the body, especially the heart, muscles, and kidneys, needs the mineral magnesium. It also contributes to the make-up and strength of our teeth and bones. "

Foods rich in magnesium include wholegrains, nuts, and green vegetables. Green leafy vegetables are particularly good sources of magnesium. Baby leaf spinach is a favourite of mine, it is easy to prepare especially if eaten raw and makes the plate look very appetising.

Vitamin D: This wonderful vitamin plays a central role in many of our body's processes and should be on the A-list for menopausal women. Studies have linked it to preventing heart disease, osteoporosis, diabetes, cancer and weight gain. Yet as many as half of all adults are deficient in vitamin D and therefore do not benefit from it. Sunblock inhibits not only UV rays but also vitamin D, and today's lifestyles and work and school habits mean that we spend most of our time indoors rather than out in the sun. Glass blocks UV rays and vitamin D and therefore it is a false presumption to believe that the window provides you with adequate nutrition. Getting out into the sun is crucial for optimising absorption of this mineral, and you do not need to lay down in it for hours on end to do this. And for the health of your skin it is important to try and expose your legs as well as your upper body to natural sunlight.

Alcohol can affect the reproductive hormones in postmenopausal women. After menopause, estradiol levels decline drastically because the hormone is no longer synthesised in the ovaries, and only small amounts are derived from the conversion of testosterone in other tissues. This estradiol deficiency has been associated with an increased risk of cardiovascular disease and osteoporosis in postmenopausal women. Alcohol can increase the conversion of testosterone into estradiol, assisting in the elevation of estradiol levels in postmenopausal women who consume alcohol, over those who abstain. And studies have shown that postmenopausal women who consume three to six drinks per week may reduce the risk of cardiovascular disease without significantly impairing bone quality or increasing the risk of alcoholic liver disease or breast cancer.

(Acknowledgement: The National Institute on Alcohol Abuse and Alcoholism - contributions of Judith Fradkin, M.D Chief, Endocrinology and Metabolic Diseases Program Branch, National Institute of Diabetes and Digestive and Kidney Diseases).

9

Asthma and the Pelvic Floor

There are many conditions that can have an adverse affect on the pelvic floor but asthma, which has its own debilitations, can also have a long-term detrimental effect.

I have included this special chapter for a very dear friend of mine, whom I am working with, and together we would like to be able to help others in this position.

The word asthma simply means 'difficulty breathing.' Approximately 5.1 million people in the UK suffer from asthma. I tell my clients that no matter what exercise they want to do, the 'breathing is everything.' The first exercise in chapter 13 is simply titled 'The Beauty of Breathing' and is also known as 'ALIVE' or the first principle of the Pelvic Floor Secrets Conditioning Program, no matter which package you choose. I believe the information written here could prove invaluable to many asthma sufferers on a number of levels:

Asthma - the condition affects the breathing tubes 'the bronchi' (the tiny tubes within the bronchus, see picture page 144), which are usually very sensitive in asthma sufferers and slightly inflamed. As these are the tubes that ultimately carry the air/oxygen to the lungs it is easy for a sufferer to experience a restriction, which can be triggered by dust and/or allergies, which get into the airways, causing what is known medically as an asthma attack.

Chapter Ten

Those who have suffered asthma since childhood and the constant cough that comes with it are usually pre-disposed to stress urinary incontinence. This is because the constant cough, discussed earlier, creates what is known as continuous "intra-abdominal" pressure – in other words a constant downward force of the internal organs on the pelvic floor muscles every time you cough. As the pelvic floor is a hidden set of muscles that is not taught or indeed talked about in mainstream education or social settings, its wellbeing is not CONSIDERED and the muscles are not conditioned as a prerequisite to offset the dysfunction that comes with a de-conditioned pelvic floor. This means the pelvic floor can become excessively weak (sometime developing tiny tears within the muscle – tissue breakdown) and thus the ability of the urethral sphincter to 'close' fully and prevent urinary loss when coughing, or any other movement including jumping, sneezing etc has become compromised. (see sketch on page 120)

> " *Those who have suffered asthma since childhood and the constant cough that comes with it are usually pre-disposed to stress urinary incontinence.* "

It is IMPERATIVE that ALL asthma sufferers are educated about the role and responsibility of their pelvic floor especially with regard to the excessive pressure their condition (asthma) exerted on their floor. It is equally important to note, that excess weight, smoking and the usual everyday activities can add to an already excessively 'overloaded' pelvic floor and that this could lead to pelvic organ prolapse – usually the bladder. When this happens many surgeons are reluctant to do repairs such as the TVT sling (see page 100) as the failure rate is too high. Again, this is because the foundation exercise is missing (not thought about or taught) and without a solid foundation, it is impossible for the 'support' that is required to 'keep' the organs in their anatomical position.

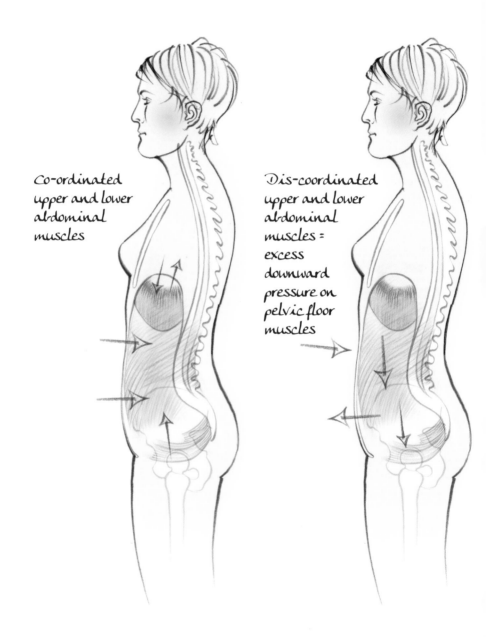

Co-ordinated upper and lower abdominal muscles

Dis-coordinated upper and lower abdominal muscles = excess downward pressure on pelvic floor muscles

A couple of years ago for my son's 15th birthday we invited some of his friends from school over for a barbecue. I love my garden hammocks and we bought a third one. This one had a more study metal frame and needed screw drivers and drills to put it together. It was more like a hammock bed – lovely. Well, everyone loved that hammock, especially in the sunshine, and on they piled... all SEVEN! It lasted not even one afternoon. It just collapsed in the middle! £170 wasted. The point I am making is the hammock was fit for purpose, but it was not designed for that excessive load and just like the sketch I put in earlier it "just could not hold them up for long."

10

Think about it. You don't need a degree for this: if a muscle is de-conditioned it is dysfunctional. In other words, muscles that do not have the right amount of conditioning and density are less likely to be able to "perform" optimally. Now when it comes to the pelvic floor – that hammock-like sling (see picture on page 56) that has the upper part of the vagina, rectum, bladder and uterus 'sitting on it' and then the organs of the viscera (intestines) etc resting above, without the support of our natural girdle – the transverse abdominals, then this poor hammock will begin to tear and then collapse which means the contents drop, allowing pain and embarrassment to jump right in.

Think of your pelvic floor in the same way as the example given and begin to regard its strength and limitations. Then you can begin to protect yourself against embarrassment and debilitation and just enjoy the pleasure it can bring.

Testicular Cancer and Prostate Issues

HAVING taught pelvic floor health for many years, I am still amazed when men say to me, "Do we have a pelvic floor?" The answer to those who do not know is a resounding YES! The pelvic floor is the foundation of the trunk, full stop, not just the female trunk alone. Its responsibility for support of the organs and voluntary elimination of urine or faeces is exactly the same, as is its role in sexual pleasure. It is here though that the pelvic floor obviously differs and therefore pelvic floor strength and conditioning is executed differently, because of the anatomy of the area. This section of the book is to encourage, educate and motivate men towards optimising their pelvic floor health. There is a reward for you also. Women, this section is also a must for you. Researching this section has been fascinating and speaking so bluntly about it has really helped me to understand testicular and prostate health, and why it is crucial for men to be aware of their pelvic floor health and understand how everything works together.

> " *The male menopause does exist, but manifests itself in more subtle ways. It is a more gradual incremental process, which begins for many men from the age of twenty. But, because it is so incremental it is barely noticeable until midlife.* "

The male menopause does exist, but manifests itself in more subtle ways. It is a more gradual incremental process, which begins for many men from the age of twenty. But, because it is so incremental it is barely noticeable until midlife.

Chapter Eleven

Some of the symptoms are; flagging energy, an increased waistline, a duller mind, less drive and ambition, sore muscles, a lowering libido, and a struggling erection. The male menopause is also known as a lowering of the male dominant hormone, testosterone. Do not cry guys, it does not necessarily mean that it will affect your sex drive. It is a change in the signals from your pituitary gland to your testes that causes the production of testosterone to lower. You can opt for testosterone replacement therapy, but it has been found that a combination of remedies is needed to treat this.

A POINT TO NOTE: ALL OVERWEIGHT MEN HAVE A LOWER-THAN-NORMAL LEVEL OF TESTOSTERONE. THIS IS BECAUSE AS THE ACCUMULATION OF FAT INCREASES, THE MANUFACTURE OF TESTOSTERONE DECREASES, AND CONVERTS SOME OF THE TESTOSTERONE TO ESTROGEN. AS YOUR ESTROGEN LEVELS RISE (ALSO A REASON WHY MEN CAN DEVELOP BREASTS), YOUR MUSCLES BECOME WEAKER AND YOUR ABILITY TO BURN FAT DECREASES. A BRISK 20 MINUTE WALK INCLUDED INTO THE WORKING DAY, CAN HELP THE WEIGHT DECREASE, AND IT DOES, SO TOO DOES THE LEVEL OF ESTROGEN, WHICH CAN IN TURN, ALLOW FOR MORE TESTOSTERONE PRODUCTION.

It is possible for a man to have a testosterone level test, measuring the levels before the age of 40 to get a good baseline. Having the levels checked bi-annually thereafter, says Dr Eugene Shippen, M.D. from Shillington, Pennyslvania, will mean men will know when their testosterone levels begin to decline.

Whenever I teach a pelvic floor masterclass I always start by saying, "For the purposes of this workshop, I am going to repeatedly ask you to either close the vaginal lips and zip up, or lift and lower your testicles from the ground floor to the penthouse! If you feel embarrassed, then you need to leave." Interestingly, when men do the exercises and realise their testicles can move they excitedly come and say things like, "You're right Jenni, my testicles can move. When I get really good I will come back and let you know." What a wonderful thing to be told. Indeed, when I taught a workshop in early 2005, I had approximately 90 people, 15 of whom were men.

In my first book *"Can a Vagina really buy a Mercedes?"* I have a section called Jimmy Choo. Out in the outback in your £2,000 Jimmy Choo shoes and needing to go to the toilet, I describe a snake being underneath you and you needing to stop the urine and stand, so you need to engage your pelvic floor and stand up without losing a drop. One sweet gentleman at the back, completely in the zone, put his hand up and said, "I can't lift my testicles!" Speechless for a moment I then shrugged my shoulders and answered, "I can't help you." The room erupted in laughter – but this is a great example of how effective it can be. He is great now though! The workshops are great fun as well as being informative – not all workshops are mixed, but it is statements like this that relax the atmosphere and allow people to open up and share their experiences.

Men, this is how you engage your pelvic floor, but you also have another part of the floor that is conditioned when you ejaculate and that is the prostate gland.

Your prostate gland is located immediately beneath the bladder (the bladder stores urine until it is emptied). It is a small cone shaped organ, usually around half an inch long, weighing less than an ounce. It encircles the base of the urethra, where it joins the bladder. The gland emits a thin and milky fluid, known as prostatic fluid. This substance enables the sperm, which comes from the testicles, to remain alive. The basic properties of prostatic fluid actually help to balance the acidic environment of the vagina and also protect the sperm from urinary traces. It also assists in stopping semen and urine from mixing together as both are discharged through the urethra.

Male pelvic floor/penis

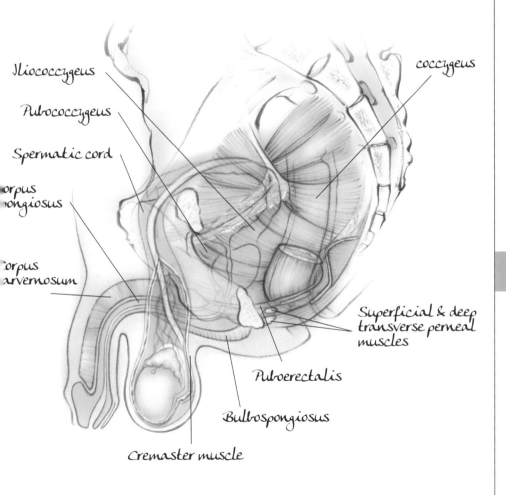

Iliococcygeus

Pubococcygeus

Spermatic cord

orpus
ongiosus

orpus
arvernosum

coccygeus

Superficial & deep
transverse perneal
muscles

Puboerectalis

Bulbospongiosus

Cremaster muscle

11

" Because of the close relationship between the prostate gland and the urinary tract, if there is a problem in one system, it can have far-reaching implications for the other. "

Because of the close relationship between the prostate gland and the urinary tract, if there is a problem in one system, it can have far-reaching implications for the other.

Under your prostate gland is a pair of smaller glands known as the bulbourethral glands, which are connected to the urethra, hence the name. Their main function is still not known, however they do secrete a fluid before ejaculation. It is believed that these glands help lubricate the penis (although they only secrete one or two drops, not believed to be enough for the whole of the penis).

On either side of the urethra just above your prostate gland lives the seminal vesicle. 55% of semen is produced here. Semen's main function is the protection of the sperm cells in the vagina. The fluid is thick and translucent, containing amino acids, fructose and mucus, all of which provide the sperms cells with energy. It also contains the lipid compound prostaglandin. Prostaglandins stimulate the uterine muscles to assist in quickening the movement of the sperm cells into the uterus, towards the eggs. Millions of sperm cells join with this fluid as they are ejected through the urethra by undulating contractions, via the prostate gland. These contractions and discharge are known as ejaculation. This is the best way to condition your prostate gland.

Your testicles and scrotum are the visual link for pelvic floor conditioning. The testicles (usually two) dangle beneath the "penis bag" of skin, which is known as the scrotum - a small walnut shaped, wrinkled bag. Each testicle is made up of tightly coiled seminiferous tubules (tiny tubes in which spermatozoa or sperm cells are formed), which manufactures more than 250 million sperm cells every day. The sperm cells are stored within the testes themselves and if they are not released, then they break down (no, they do not cry!) and are absorbed into the bloodstream. There are interstitial cells within the testicles (cells in-between the seminiferous tubules) which produce testosterone, the steroid hormone responsible for your sexual urges.

A fact to note, men: Your sperm needs to be maintained at a temperature that is 2C less than your interior body temperature and thus scientists believe this is why your testicles are in their vulnerable position outside of the body.

When required the muscle fibres within the scrotum contract and elevate the testicles towards the body to help keep them warm (because of the sperm), and relaxes and lowers them away when it gets too warm.

The testicles originate in the abdomen. The layers of tissue that enclose each testicle are derived from layers of the anterior abdominal wall. The muscle that is responsible for drawing the testicles up towards the body and then relaxing them is known as the cremasteric muscle, which arises from the internal oblique muscle. The cremasteric muscle is a part of the spermatic cord, a pair of tubular structures that support the testes in the scrotum. This is the first section through which your sperm passes before ejaculation. As this muscle contracts, the spermatic cord is shortened and this allows the testicles to move closer to the body in a bid to provide a little more warmth to the delicate sperm cells. The opposite then happens as the testicles are lowered away from the body and the temperature becomes too warm. It is

> " A fact to note, men: Your sperm needs to be maintained at a temperature that is 2C less than your interior body temperature and thus scientists believe this is why your testicles are in their vulnerable position outside of the body. "

known as the cremasteric reflex. This action also happens in response to stress, with the testicles moving up towards your body as a means of protection. It is believed that there is a relaxation of the testicles as you approach orgasm and then a retraction during the orgasm itself.

Your pubococcygeus muscle (PC) in the pelvic floor (also known as the love muscle of the pelvic floor) is attached to the pubic bone in front and the coccyx (tailbone) at the back, forming part of the pelvic floor (platform). This floor is a hammock-like sling at the base of the pelvic cavity, and has a partial responsibility in the activation of the testicles, playing an important role in ejaculation, along with the testes and prostate gland.

Conditioning the Pubococcygeus (PC) has some amazing benefits for men:

◆ Stronger and firmer erections
◆ Ability to fully control penile movement during intercourse (able to bounce up and down)
◆ Ability to offset ejaculation
◆ Stronger and more intense orgasms
◆ Ability to "shoot" – ejaculate further
◆ Optimised urinary health

During orgasm the PC muscle contracts and relaxes in a rhythmic fashion. It is part of a system of muscles that propels semen from the body (along with the prostate, perineal muscle and penis shaft). This is the "reward" for strengthening these muscles.

Orgasms feel far more pleasurable and ejaculation distance is increased. Whilst the PC muscle is only one part of the ejaculatory system, it is a major part.

Many male porn stars condition their PC muscles daily in order to ensure their ejaculation distance – the "cumshots" or "moneyshots" as they are known, are more impressive.

> *A POINT TO NOTE:* ALTHOUGH YOUR PC MUSCLE CAN INCREASE YOUR EJACULATION DISTANCE / STRENGTH, IT CANNOT INCREASE SEMEN VOLUME, AS THE PC IS NOT INVOLVED IN THE PRODUCTION OF SEMEN.

> 66 *Many male porn stars condition their PC muscles daily in order to ensure their ejaculation distance – the "cumshots" or "moneyshots" as they are known, are more impressive.* 99

The exercises in Chapter 13 are unisex and are activated in the same way for both men and women. It is just the identification (through the testes for men as opposed to through the vagina for women) that makes it different, but strengthens the PC muscles in the same way. You now have a little more information about the most precious part of your body. Understanding and optimising pelvic floor health can also help to offset two of the biggest cancers for men, testicular and prostate. Read the information below, apply the advice, and by the grace of God you will have optimal pelvic floor health and another reason for continuing to make love to your wife at least 3 times per week for anyone under sixty, and at least once for the over sixties, according to the medical experts!

Hard Flaccid Penis

Hard Flaccid Penis is a vascular condition of the penis that causes the smooth muscles of the Corpora Cavernosa (the two chambers that run the length of the penis, filled with spongy tissue, which fills with blood in the open spaces to create an erection) to suddenly remain in a chronic state of contraction and/or tension. This causes decreased / abnormal blood flow, numbness, pain and erectile dysfunction. It usually occurs immediately after a mild injury or trauma (including

11

increased levels of stress), but can also present idiopathically (of unknown cause) or gradually.

It presents as hard or firm to the touch, but not erect or enlarged in any way. Unlike other penile dysfunction, it is not systemic, meaning that it does not affect the whole body and thus can be alleviated by either lying down or positions the body to cause the muscles to relax (on all fours may help with the gravitational pull). The onset of hard flaccid penis is immediate, pronounced veins, which distinguish it from other well-known penile conditions. Many men experience this around increased stress in their personal lives, which can have detrimental affects on sexual function – the body sacrificing the sex and repair hormones, for your stress hormones. It can be a very debilitating dysfunction that affects men not just physically but emotionally also. Pelvic floor exercises, as mentioned above, increases the blood flow to the area and can help to relieve this condition. It is good to seek help from a physical therapist also, in conjunction with or outside of the exercises in this book. (Look in the reference guide at the back of the book)

Testicular Cancer

This is a rare type of cancer that appears to be on the increase. It is more prevalent in black men aged 15-45 and also among middle class Caucasians. No one is certain about the causes, but there are some certain risk factors. If a close family member has been diagnosed with the disease then your risk of being diagnosed is increased. Furthermore, if one or both of a boy's testicles have not descended by around the age of seven (approximately) then his risk of developing the disease is greatly increased in later life.

There are four distinct early warning signs, which are usually easy to spot:

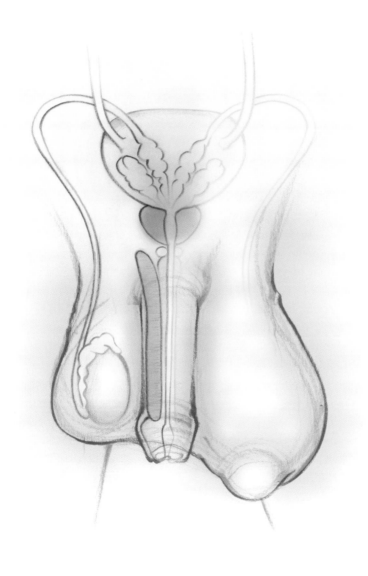

1. A hard lump on the front or side of the testicle
2. An enlargement or swelling of a testicle
3. Pain or discomfort in a testicle or in the scrotum
4. An unusual difference between the two testicles

This is why it is important that young boys are taught how to check themselves as they enter into puberty. It is very easy to check yourself and the best time to do this is either in the shower or bath, or immediately after you get out. Since we are all different, it is important that we get to know ourselves better than anyone else knows us, so we can gauge what is normal or abnormal. Hold your scrotum in the palm of your hand and feel the size and weight of your testicles. If, in subsequent checks, the weight is heavier than usual then visit your doctor. Remember it is normal to have one testicle larger than the other and one that hangs lower than the other. You should roll each testicle between your thumb and finger. It should feel smooth. If it doesn't, you should make an appointment to see your doctor but you should also remember that there are other causes for changes in your testicles. It is unusual to develop testicular cancer in both testicles at the same time, so ensure that you compare one with the other.

Testicular cancer is almost always curable if discovered early and even if it has spread to other parts of your body, it does respond well to treatment, and the good news is that nine out of ten sufferers are cured and continue to enjoy a normal sex life and go on to successfully father children.

Prostate Issues

The prostate gland, situated immediately beneath the bladder, is nature's way of ensuring the continuation of the human race. This walnut sized gland provides most of the fluid (semen) in which the male sperm travels, on its way to the female egg so that fertilisation can take place. Nature, however, has played a trick on men, in that the urethra, the tube through which urine passes from the bladder to exit the body via the penis, passes through the prostate. When a man is young and his prostate healthy this process of elimination works fine, but as man begins to age, there is a tendency for things to go wrong.

There are three main issues with regard to prostate health:

1. Prostatitis is the least severe of the issues relating to prostate health and falls into two classes; acute and chronic.

> a. Acute prostatitis is usually caused by a virus or bacteria and has symptoms similar to VD or gonorrhoea. Treatment is usually with antibiotics and the sufferer can return to their normal daily activities after a short period of time.

> b. Chronic prostatitis however, is a different kettle of fish. The word "chronic" tells us that this is an ongoing scenario. This condition manifests itself with bouts of impotence, which can last anything from one week to many years, with the sufferer experiencing periods of sexual normality followed by periods of erectile dysfunction. It is almost an oxymoron, but stress will/can prolong periods of impotency.

> Since no one knows the cause of prostatitis, no one has come up with a cure.

2. Benign Prostatic Hyperplasia (Hypertrophy - BPH) is the most common prostate ailment afflicting men, and manifests itself in many ways. Fungal infections are a very common cause of BPH and prostate

11

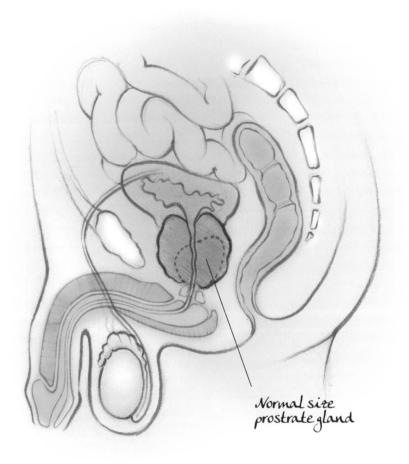

Normal size
prostrate gland

cancer. Reference: Doug Kaufmann *'The Germ that causes Cancer.'* As the name implies this is a non-cancerous enlargement of the prostate, which is common as men get older. The symptoms of BPH are:

◆ A weak stream of urine
◆ Dribbling
◆ Inability or delay in the start of urination
◆ Urgency (when you want to go - you have to go)
◆ Erectile dysfunction

It would seem that Mother Nature continues to play her tricks on many men, in that they can have all or some of the symptoms of BPH, yet not have prostate cancer and conversely they can have no symptoms of BPH but can have prostate cancer, a signal of its complexity and the importance of being properly diagnosed.

There is an accepted method of testing for prostate cancer, by way of a Prostate Specific Antigen (PSA) blood test, in conjunction with a Digital Rectal Examination (DRE). (PSA is a prostate specific protein found in the prostate gland produced as a result of fungal mycotoxins. See reference for Doug Kaufmann at back of book)

A sample of blood is taken and then sent to a lab where tests are carried out to measure the amount of prostatic protein in the bloodstream. Cancerous cells also produce this protein but in an elevated amount compared to normal cells. A reading is then assessed and measured in ng/ml. A prostatic protein reading of 4ng/ml is considered normal whereas any reading between 4ng/ml and 10ng/ml could indicate the presence of cancer, and a reading above 10 is considered a strong indicator of cancer. However, there are certain factors, besides cancer, that can cause an elevated PSA reading,

11

namely, infection, BPH, having had sex within 72 hours of having the PSA test, and having had a DRE; these can all be false indicators.

A Digital Rectal Examination, DRE, involves the insertion of a gloved finger into the rectal passage in order to feel the prostate gland. The doctor will be looking for the presence of any lumps or hardness, as these usually imply that there is cancer present. This invasive procedure tends to put men off ensuring the health of their prostate and thus preventing health problems later on. The DRE, when combined with the PSA blood test, has been the main yardstick for diagnosing prostate cancer for many years. Unfortunately, there have been many instances of misdiagnosis that have resulted in a number of men having their prostate glands removed prematurely. These "false positives" as they are called, have resulted in the PSA blood test being called into question with regard to its accuracy or lack thereof. The consensus therefore is to always get a second opinion from a prostate specialist.

HUMOUR: An old man of 68 years, visits his doctors for a DRE, but his usual doctor was not available. Instead a beautiful and curvaceous woman is in his place. "Please lay on your tummy, Sir" she asks the man, "so that I can insert my finger to investigate your prostate." She asks him to say 99 when he can feel her! She then asks him to turn on his side and finally his back. "Because of the nature of your anatomy I need to support your penis in my left hand whilst investigating one more time. Please say 99 when you can feel it." He replies, "One, two..."

Sometimes a GP may recommend a biopsy. This procedure involves the insertion of a needle into the prostate gland and a small sample of tissue taken and sent to a lab for testing. It has been reported that this procedure has a downside, in that in about 40% of the cases where a biopsy is carried out and no cancer is found, those men eventually go on to develop cancer as a result of the biopsy. It is recommended therefore, that an ultrasound scan be employed instead.

> " *Prostate cancer is considered to be a slow growing cancer and most experts say you are more likely to die with it than from it and so a system of "watchful waiting" is engaged.* "

In the unfortunate event of prostate cancer being diagnosed there are certain options available.

Prostate cancer is considered to be a slow growing cancer and most experts say you are more likely to die with it than from it and so a system of "watchful waiting" is engaged.

The cancer is checked regularly to see the rate of development. Alternatively, surgery may be employed either by way of radiation, radical prostatectomy and more recently cryosurgery.

◆ Radiation involves "seeding" the tumour with radioactive pellets. This procedure is less invasive but more expensive than surgery, and can come with adverse side effects including rectal pain, diarrhoea, incontinence and impotence

◆ Prostatectomy involves the complete removal of the prostate gland and can have the same adverse side effects as radiation

◆ Cryosurgery is a much newer technique and involves targeting cancerous cells with liquid oxygen or argon gas. It is

11

not as invasive as radiation or a prostatectomy and comes with fewer adverse side effects, and it is said that there is an 85% chance of retaining your sexual potency

Since we believe that prevention is better than cure, let us look at some lifestyle and dietary changes that can be implemented to mitigate the risk of BPH or prostate cancer itself.

Whilst recent legislation does not permit holistic health to claim its effectiveness in contributing to prostate health, there are certain foods, herbs and minerals worth including in your diet:

◆ Sweet potato, especially the orange coloured one, is full of beta-carotene, which gives it its colour. When eaten this converts into vitamin A which is not only good for night vision but also for the prostate. Incidentally, sweet potato is now considered to be one of the top 5 health foods in the world

◆ Lycopene (from tomatoes, watermelon, Spanish onions and grapefruit) is what gives these fruit and veg their reddish colour. The redder the tomato (the main source) the more lycopene, and if eaten cooked and with pepper, the body absorbs more of the lycopene

◆ Quercetin is found in broccoli, cauliflower and blueberries and is said to be very beneficial to the prostate. In fact, one report (PubMed, Feb 2011) stated that like zinc, which is also very important to prostate health, most of the lycopene found in the body is concentrated in the prostate. Recently it has been suggested that tomatoes and broccoli work better when paired together. So eating broccoli with cooked tomatoes and a little pepper is considered more beneficial than eating them separately

◆ Zinc is one of the most important minerals when it comes to prostate health as it provides an alkaline environment that protects and strengthens the sperm – all cancers live in increased acidity. Spinach is an excellent source of zinc and also contributes to fertilisation and the strengthening of sperm

◆ Selenium is a trace mineral also associated with prostate health

◆ Vitamin C and Vitamin A, and of late, Vitamin D are also considered to be extremely prostate friendly

◆ Turmeric is a very active ingredient in Ayurvedic medicine and is seen as a "cleanser of the body" and widely considered as a key ingredient in preventing prostate cancer. It has increasing anti-inflammatory properties.

Pairing of turmeric and cauliflower is said to bring out the best of both of them.

Needless to say, smoking and excess drinking of alcohol, together with some prescribed medicines impact negatively on the health of the prostate.

I had a wonderful conversation with a few of my girlfriends and told them about this chapter and what I had discovered whilst doing my research. One of my girlfriends of the same persuasion as myself asked,

11

66 *Needless to say, smoking and excess drinking of alcohol, together with some prescribed medicines impact negatively on the health of the prostate.* 99

"If the prostate is conditioned during sex, how come so many of our brothers are suffering from prostate cancer? I thought that black men were bonking away like crazy?" Take this as tongue in cheek, guys, and do not get offended!

A POINT TO NOTE: TO BONK REGULARLY REQUIRES A HIGH LEVEL OF TESTOSTERONE AND AN EXCESSIVE AMOUNT OF THIS IS ALSO LINKED TO PROSTATE CANCER. SO ALTHOUGH BONKING IS GOOD FOR EXERCISING THE PROSTATE GLAND ITSELF, THE RESULTING HIGH LEVEL OF TESTOSTERONE CAN ADVERSELY AFFECT IT. ALSO, AS MEN GET OLDER THEIR LEVEL OF TESTOSTERONE DROPS OFF WHILST THEIR LEVELS OF ESTROGEN INCREASE. THIS IS FURTHER EXACERBATED BY THE HORMONES IN DAIRY PRODUCTS, MAKING THIS COMBINATION NOT SO PROSTATE FRIENDLY.

As you can see from the list above there are foods that can help condition the prostate and this list shows a snippet of just how important your diet is to prostate health. I cannot say this enough, you are what you eat, drink, think and sleep!

A POINT TO NOTE:

- DRINKING PASTEURISED MILK REGULARLY DOUBLES YOUR RISK OF GETTING PROSTATE CANCER
- EATING COMMERCIALLY FARMED RED MEAT EVERY DAY TRIPLES THE RISK OF GETTING PROSTATE CANCER
- NOT EATING ORGANIC VEGETABLES QUADRUPLES THE RISK OF GETTING PROSTATE CANCER

I know many men who do not like to drink water either as a form of hydration or as a beverage. They choose to drink fruit juice, which equals sugar. The best solution for Pollution is Dilution says Dr Rober Rakowski D.C (clinical director of the National Medical Centre, Houston Texas). Water is nature's best most natural solvent!

A friend's relative suffered a stroke last year and now drinks plenty of water. It is an example of how we react after the damage is done. As stated previously, there are two things that we cannot buy: time and health. Here is an extract from one of my poems about time:

Time the most precious gift that God gave us all, is a gift taken lightly, with barely a thought.
Not for resale, washed away on a whim, then chased after frantic when the darkness sets in.
Use your time wisely, treasure it well –
for the moment it leaves you – you leave here as well!

The rule of thumb according to Paul Chek (HTEM BBH) for optimal health is an application towards a healthy lifestyle ratio of 80%-20%. This allows you to have one fifth of your life full of indulgence and this is a reasonable amount. It is what is known in laymen's terms as moderation. If you are not a lover of vegetables or certain foods, your prostate and testicles are, so begin to include them. Use the breathing exercises. As I always say, "The breathing is everything." Oxygen is your cells' most crucial food and diaphragmatic breathing ensures that there is a good blood flow into this most precious area of your body, helping to continue good health.

Do not be frightened of water. Understand the necessity of sleep times and try to meditate even once a week, just to clear your headspace. There is so much negativity being fed to us through the media that a 20 minute downtime, to "clear out" the rubbish and leave the brain fresh can help to regulate blood pressure and shrink stress levels. Your body will sacrifice your repair hormones and your sex hormones for your stress hormones, so if you are finding that you have erection issues, or problems maintaining an erection or even premature ejaculation, then take a 20 minute meditation session and reflect on the dominant thought processes that are occupying your head. You may just find your body fighting itself to rid you of unnecessary clutter.

11

Love Life or Love Food?

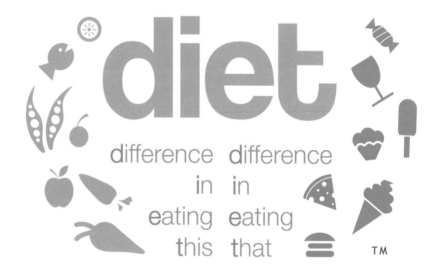

diet
difference in eating this   difference in eating that ™

WHATEVER we choose to eat, this is our diet. Whether it is a diet of beer, cigarettes and fast food, or a diet rich in organic and free-range food and quality, bottled water; our daily diet is whatever we choose for it to be. The difference is whether we choose to eat like this or to eat like that. The difference being, eating towards optimal health, or ill health. Considering the rule of thumb is an 80% - 20% ratio of healthy eating vs. indulgence, with all the information available, it is actually sinful that the majority of our nation is suffering from malnutrition of the obese kind.

Obesity is not because of good food choice or lack of access to it. It is not because life has made it impossible for us to move, because many buildings are on multi levels, the country is very undulating; there are infinite parks, fields and woods and there are also thousands of private and public health clubs and training facilities. Not to mention that Nintendo has made a mint from the sale of the Wii Fit, and now too there is an equivalent on the Xbox 360, home DVDs, equipment on teleshopping – there has never been such a great push towards a healthy lifestyle approach, and yet the NHS spends millions per minute trying to save and then educate the nation towards better life choices that can provide optimal health.

Popular English soaps are based around the pub, and pub food and takeaways are the second most popular shops on the high streets of more deprived areas, next to the bookies. I joke, tongue in cheek, that Waitrose only opens where there is money so I know my area is good!

With the availability of cheap food on the high street and the ever-present price wars between supermarkets catering for the masses, quality is not the primary consideration, and neither is sufficient nutritional value.

Salts and all kinds of crazy additives are needed to make half of these non-foods taste like food, and with the cost of food rocketing, but wages decreasing in real terms, it makes it almost impossible to get people to make the change. Ill health is a slow hidden process that manifests itself on the inside before the real symptoms begin to stop you in your tracks. By this time, for many it can be too late.

We only chase after health when it threatens to disable us or shorten our time on earth, but alarmingly,

> ❝ With the availability of cheap food on the high street and the ever-present price wars between supermarkets catering for the masses, quality is not the primary consideration, and neither is sufficient nutritional value. ❞

for many the old habits return when they feel that they are better. How can you believe you are better if you have had any part of your insides removed, if you have to endure months of chemotherapy or radiotherapy? Once your body has been through that much medical abuse, if you do not understand the importance of neutralising your system you really are not well! Chemotherapy destroys everything in its wake and that includes your immune system – the very system you need to fight all infection and free radical damage which can cause you to become very unwell very easily with no immune system available to fight with. Indeed it is impossible for any patient to undertake each chemotherapy session without first signing the consent form acknowledging the possibility that every conceivable side effect could become a reality of the treatment; crazy! I witnessed my father do this in his hope to 'cling onto life.'

It is important for you to understand what metabolism is and how your body metabolises (uses/burns) food. Think of a light bulb or even your electrical appliances. All of these have an energy efficiency rating, and so too do our bodies. The more energy efficient the body, the better it is at utilising the food and the less likely it is to have weight issues. Many people eat all the wrong foods and just say they have not got a fast metabolism, without even understanding metabolic rates and the appropriate foods to eat according to the rate at which the body burns/ utilises the food it is given. It is important also to understand what the glycaemic index (GI) means in relation to your health.

The higher the GI number of the food we consume, the faster that food can convert to sugar within the body, spiking an insulin response from the pancreas. Illnesses such as diabetes can claim the lives of around 24 million people per year (according to new research out Dec, 2011, GP Online) and the biggest at risk group is young women aged 15-24 years.

Contrary to popular belief, insulin is not a weight gaining hormone; it is a hormone responsible for food, or more specifically, glucose management.

Lack of movement, whether at work, home or through exercise, adopting a sedentary lifestyle, lack of sleep and water, and stressful thoughts, are all major culprits! Look at Halle Berry – beautiful to look at and with an amazing body, even as she matures so gracefully. She was diagnosed with type II diabetes in 1989, passing out on TV and spending a week in a diabetic coma. She took the tough words from the doctors and made the right decision to investigate the foods that would not only keep her alive but would allow her to manage her energy conversion rate (sugar levels) and weight. She is an amazing example – it is only convenience foods' dominance in our life that has allowed us to conveniently forget/ignore the primary purpose of our food, which is to nourish and feed our cells so that we can move and be healthy. We have instead made the primary purpose indulgence and enjoyment, and whilst these are important, they should not be the central focus. It is also important for a woman to understand her fat cells. Women have more fat-storing enzymes in their fat cells than men. This is because of their reproductive organs; women need the extra insulation and protection around this important area in preparation for motherhood. Fat cells tend to report for duty as the metabolism clocks off. The metabolism is optimal between 6am and 6pm, whilst our fat cells are optimal between 6pm and 6am! What time do you eat your biggest meal and then what do you do afterwards? For most women the answer is late evening after work, or once the kids have gone to bed, or having waited for your husband or partner to get home. Any activity after this is usually minimal, with no real energy expenditure, the food rests and the fat cells "interview and recruit" almost instantly.

12

66 *If you want to see whether you would lose a few pounds, reverse your food for a week – dinner for breakfast and breakfast for dinner!* 99

If you want to see whether you would lose a few pounds, reverse your food for a week – dinner for breakfast and breakfast for dinner!

For more information on this subject, read *Outsmarting the Female Fat Cell* by Debra Waterhouse. Dieting actually encourages active growth of the fat cell through the famine/feast principle, and our fat cells can increase by up to 50% of their original size – so when you return to normal eating habits your body returns to extra expansion. There is not a quick fix, ladies - I have seen and worked with women who have had liposuction and then ended up 1.5 times the size they were in the first place. A good body requires your undivided attention and that means knowing and understanding how YOUR body works, what it likes and how it responds to food, water, sleep, exercise, digestion, elimination, load and stress etcetera.

A POINT TO NOTE: THE ILLNESS DIABETES IS A DYSFUNCTION OF THE BODY'S INABILITY TO USE GLUCOSE AS IT SHOULD. EXCESS GLUCOSE IN THE BLOOD CAN ACT AS A POISON, AND IT IS THIS POISON THAT CAN DAMAGE THE NEPHRONS WITHIN THE KIDNEYS AND LEAD TO DIABETIC KIDNEY DISEASE. MANY DIABETIC SUFFERERS ALSO DEVELOP HIGH BLOOD PRESSURE, ANOTHER DYSFUNCTION THAT CAN DAMAGE THE SMALL BLOOD VESSELS WITHIN THE KIDNEYS. IF YOU FIND YOURSELF SUFFERING FROM EITHER OF THESE TWO ILLNESSES YOU SHOULD SEEK THE HELP OF A LEVEL 3 CHEK HLC COACH (WWW.BODYCHEK.COM).

Going back to diabetes; when we eat foods that convert quickly to sugar, the pancreas, which is responsible for regulating the amount of sugar that gets into our bloodstream, releases the hormone insulin in order to regulate the flow of and control of sugar. The pancreas actually completes the job of breaking down proteins, carbohydrates and fats, using digestive juices and juices from the intestines. But it is not only insulin that is produced here. Glucagon is another hormone produced by the pancreas that raises the levels of (sugar) glucose in the blood.

Pelvic Floor Secrets

Insulin stimulates the cells to use the glucose and somatostatin helps to regulate the secretion of these two hormones. The pancreas also produces chemicals that neutralise stomach acids, which pass from the stomach into the small intestine by using substances within the pancreatic juice.

By better understanding the hormones released by the pancreas; raising blood sugar levels and then fighting to regulate them, it might just help us to realise how easy it is over time for the pancreas to become overworked and dysfunctional, especially if we pay no attention, and this is just one of the many vital organs. The pancreas also affects the types of stool we produce and the types of stool we produce can affect continence. So there is no getting away from the kinetic chain that has a knock on effect if we continue to pay no attention.

> " *In our quest to stay slim we are eliminating the fat from our diet, without realising the difference between the fats that will help to make us slim, and the fats that will help to make us fat.* "

The quick release of sugar gives us instant energy. As the body starts to work to control the levels of sugar we feel full of life, but that is short lived, and many people get what is known as energy highs and lows, where they feel full of life one minute and then tired and lethargic the next. What makes it worse is in our quest to stay slim we are eliminating the fat from our diet, without realising the difference between the fats that will help to make us slim, and the fats that will help to make us fat. "

Fat is an essential part of everybody's diet. The right fats eaten in proportion to the protein on our plates will:

◆ Help the body better breakdown the protein for digestion and distribution on for nutrition

12

◆ Slow down the rate at which the body turns carbohydrates, GI foods, into sugar

Unlike the many diets that tell you fat is bad, fat is crucial for the efficient metabolism of all protein and for weight management. Saturated fats are the best types but there are variations in the quality. It is also important to be aware that coconut oil is the best oil for cooking, as it is one of the very few that does not breakdown under high heat. Olive oil is great for dressing – but SHOULD NOT be used for cooking.

◆ Fat is an essential part of any balanced diet. It provides the body with the fat-soluble vitamins A, D, E and K, which are essential for growth. It contains essential fatty acids, which are important in maintaining normal health and body functions

◆ Although animal fats are often considered to be 'bad fats', goose fat is one of the better ones and contains far fewer saturated fats than butter or lard. Goose fat contains 32.7g saturated fat per 100g compared with 54g for butter and 40.8g for lard

◆ Goose fat is high in 'heart healthy' monounsaturated fats (55g per 100g compared to 19.8g in 100g of butter) and polyunsaturated fats (10.8g per 100g compared to 2.6g in 100g of butter)

◆ Goose fat is also rich in Oleic acid C18.1 (an omega 9 monounsaturated fatty acid), which can lower blood cholesterol levels, promoting HDLs (good cholesterol), slowing the development of heart disease, and promoting the production of antioxidants. Goose fat contains on average, 58% oleic acid

C18.1 and is generally higher in comparison to other animal fats, and potatoes roasted in goose fat are amazing!

The National Institute of Health reports that supplements containing medium-chain triglycerides may be used during cancer treatment. This is because patients with cancer may not be able to digest fat in their diet. As a result, alternative sources of healthy fat are required. Since medium-chain triglycerides are soluble in water and more readily absorbed by the body than longer-chain molecules, these are the focus for patients with cancer. Today they can be found in supplemental form.

Coconut Oil

This is the best oil to cook with, especially at high temperatures. This is because it does not become unstable with heat and therefore does not release the transfats that many other oils do when they reach the same heat. According to the Mayo Clinic, coconut oil is a good source of medium-chain triglycerides, or MCT, a triglyceride with a fatty acid chain length of six to ten carbon atoms. It is important to know the chain length and its reaction in water, according to a 2010 study in the *International Journal of Food Sciences and Nutrition,* as this determines its susceptibility to being stored in the fat tissue. The chain length in coconut oil makes it more soluble in water, meaning that it is less susceptible to being stored in the adipose (fat) tissue. This research was undertaken primarily to determine the benefits in relation to health and exercise.

12

A report in *Medical News Today* (Sep, 2009), states that when you consume coconut oil, it is not stored in the fat cells and may boost metabolism. This report also states that unlike long-chain triglycerides, this source of triglycerides may promote weight loss and prevent obesity. Whilst this may be seen as a cosmetic finding, it is a good place to start in the quest for a healthier, leaner lifestyle.

By understanding or acquiring the information about the different types of fat and the ones that are beneficial, you no longer remove it from your diet. Instead, enjoy it in its natural form and see your health go from strength to strength and your weight normalise.

In just the same way as we need to learn everything about our job in order to be able to excel and climb the business ladder, so too should we understand our health.

In every other area of our life we seem willing to do 'whatever it takes' to succeed, except in the area of our health. I heard a dear lady on a radio talk show this morning, talking about how her husband found out he had diabetes and made the changes because he told his wife, "If I want to live I have to do what the doctor tells me," and her moral of the story was, "If you want to live you must do as you are told," although she admitted she could not do it. I find this to be true of many households and it is sad.

There is a health scare for one family member and it is diet and lifestyle related, so in order to love life, that member makes a change. Why then wouldn't you think that his/her bad eating habits, the same habits you have, might also produce a health risk for you or another family member also? We have all the resources in the form of food and open space to keep us fit and healthy; why do we need the pills made up by a pharmaceutical company to keep us going? Maybe if there were a better understanding of oxidation, the speed at which food is converted to energy, people would be able to make the right food choices to stop them from gaining weight, stressing organs and joints, and putting their

> ❝ In just the same way as we need to learn everything about our job in order to be able to excel and climb the business ladder, so too should we understand our health. ❞

health in harm's way. It is sad that the choice really does come down to *'love life or love food!'* when it should be *'love life AND love food!'*

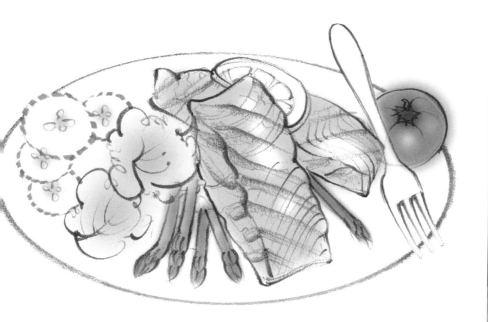

Metabolism and the Metabolic Typing® Diet

As a great colleague and friend Warren Williams (Integrated Health Coaching – www.warrenwilliamscoaching.com) says, diet is individual and cultural. However, the Western diet does have a lot to answer for with the refined produce which dominates over the organically grown food many of our fore-parents, planted and harvested. Metabolic Typing® (*The Metabolic Typing Diet* (Doubleday, 2000), by William L Wolcott) is a science, and whilst it may seem complex, it is no more complex than our genetic make-up and thus, if we begin to understand ourselves better, by sensing our reactions to foods, knowing our Metabolic Type® and dominant pathway within our own body, we are better prepared and able to combat degenerative disease and whatever the environment and life throws at us. Whilst we do have choices, a diet right for our Metabolic Type® is definitely one worth considering.

Metabolism is the name given to the chemical reactions within the body that take place in order for us to live, including the breakdown of food into energy; energy conversion. This process, the conversion of carbohydrates, proteins and fats into energy is known as oxidation. The official definition for Metabolic Typing® is: The specific, systematic, testable, repeatable and verifiable technology needed to:

Determine one's Metabolic Type®
The sum total pattern of all genetically-based strengths and weaknesses as expressed through the myriad of physical (external and internal),

psychological (mental, emotional, personality), diet-related, and functional characteristics that define biological individuality and thereby dictate nutritional requirements and therapeutic protocols

- ◆ Achieve biochemical balance
- ◆ Maximise metabolic efficiency
- ◆ Restore functional efficiency
- ◆ Produce peak performance
- ◆ Obtain optimal health
- ◆ Unfold full genetic potential

Metabolic Typing® actually involves analysis of 11 Fundamental Homeostatic Controls as well as determination and eradication of ALL possible stressors and blocking factors, internally and externally, in one's lifestyle. I strongly advise and recommend that you read *The Metabolic Typing Diet* by William L. Wolcott. As you can see, our bodies are not a one size fits all and thus to determine our reactions to our foods, environment, lifestyle etc, cannot ever be as simple as the adverts try and lead us to believe.

There are two pathways that determine how/when food is converted, and assist the body to maintain its optimal pH balance (also known as the body's chemistry). By determining a person's MetabolicType®, a diet based on optimal energy conversion is recommended, subsequently the individual can fine-tune this diet to optimise wellbeing, normalise weight, increase energy levels and offset ill health.

The oxidative and autonomic nervous systems both relate to the creation, maintenance and control of energy and both are directly stimulated or inhibited by the foods we eat. Thus the foods we eat, the food groups and food portions are very much individual, and in order to achieve and/or ensure optimal health, our body should never be reliant on one foodstuff (rotate foods and food groups) and neither too acidic, nor too alkaline all the time. Our bodies should actually cycle acid and alkaline twice in a 24 hour period, to ensure that it does not find itself in defense against a degenerative process or the presence of one, that will lead to disease. This cycle is an indication of health! (Ref: *The Metabolic Typing Diet*, William L Woolcott). This can be very hard to achieve as we live in a very acidic environment, with contributors to this being:

◆ Our levels of stress
◆ The amount of processed or ready-made food consumed
◆ Alcohol consumed
◆ Cigarettes smoked
◆ The quality of the water we drink
◆ Cookware used
◆ Neon lights from products left on standby in our bedrooms, which includes our mobile telephones

Today's diet is also made up of white (refined) bread, rice, potatoes, pasta and many convenient pre-packaged 'unnatural' foods and drinks. All of these foods have a high glycaemic index and the higher the index (which measures the rate at which a foodstuff is easily converted into sugars) the faster the surge in sugar and the more overworked the pancreas, amongst other organs, can become. The health food agency tells us to eat our five a day of fruit and vegetables, assuming that everybody oxidises food at exactly the same rate. But if we continue to eat white rice over wholegrain, white breads over wholegrain, and white potato over sweet potato, for example, then we are eating the variations of these foodstuffs that convert quickly into sugars. In doing so we are creating what are known as 'insulin spikes'. The mistake that many people make when they cut out sugar is to increase their intake of fruits, which are natural sugars, simple enough to get into the bloodstream very quickly.

Oxidation Rate refers to the speed/rate at which a person metabolises (burns/converts) carbohydrates into energy. People that are classed as Protein Types, usually burn carbohydrates at an accelerated rate and in order for them to not continually experience insulin spikes, by eating the wrong foods and "burning" it too quickly. They are better suited to a diet that is made up of more dense/dark meats and fish and higher levels of "good" fats to help assimilate the protein they have just eaten, as the rate of conversion suits their genetic make-up and they require less vegetables = carbohydrates. A person who converts carbohydrates at a slower rate (Carbohydrate Type), requires or is better suited to a diet of lighter (white) meats and fish, with less fat and is able to eat a larger portion of carbohydrate (low, medium and high starch) than their Protein counterpart.

> " Type II diabetes is a lifestyle induced illness, where the pancreas is no longer able to regulate the sugars within the system. Put simply, this is usually as a result of constant 'insulin spikes and drops' "

Type II diabetes is a lifestyle induced illness, where the pancreas is no longer able to regulate the sugars within the system. Put simply, this is usually as a result of constant 'insulin spikes and drops' caused by the food being consumed. Many Type II diabetics are slow oxidisers, so it is crucial for them to understand that vegetables are carbohydrates, with differing levels of starch. It is the levels of starch that determine their conversion rates and thus many high starch foods are cleverly referred to as "caution carbs" in the Metabolic Typing® Plan.

13

By eating according to your Metabolic Type® you can begin to optimise your health and also understand food groups and their impact on you as an individual. Yes, it may mean cooking different foods for mealtimes, but if we utilise the food differently but all eat the same, not everyone is going to benefit in the long run.

Food groups on the portion wheels below are broken into two groups, Eyes and No Eyes:

Eyes are defined as foods from animal sources and are listed as proteins and fats
◆ Cows – Beef & Dairy
◆ Pigs – Bacon, Pork, Ham
◆ Goats & Lambs – Meat
◆ Chickens & Ducks – Meat, Eggs
◆ Shrimp – Meat
◆ Fishes – Meat

No Eyes is defined as non-animal sources:
◆ Fruits
◆ Vegetables
◆ Legumes
◆ Grains

Exceptions are the following, because of their high fat content.
◆ Avocados
◆ Seeds
◆ Nuts

Reference Paul Chek; *How to Eat, Move and Be Healthy 2004.*
There are three metabolic types according to the plan:

Protein Types – are also known as Parasympathetics or Fast Oxidisers, which means that they burn food relatively quickly and thus need more

dense food - dark meats and
dark fish, with relatively little green
vegetables and barely any fruit to
slow down their oxidative rate. This
is in complete contrast to the
advertised eating habits by health
agencies. Protein types also do well on
raw nuts such as almonds, walnuts and cashews,
and full fat rich/heavy desserts such as natural yoghurt
and high quality goats and feta cheese for example.

Protein types, dependent on the dominant systems (oxidative
or autonomic) are either more acidic (oxidative) or alkaline
(parasympathetic) and thus their food behaves completely differently.
In a fast oxidiser dominant protein type, meat is akalinising and
carbohydrates acidifying, which is the complete opposite for a protein
type who is parasympathetic dominant. Whilst protein types do better
on a diet of up to 45% of protein on their plate, with approximately 20%
fats and 35% carbohydrates, they must find their own macronutrient
ratio and this requires you to pay attention to your body's reactions
to the food you have consumed. A headache shortly after eating can
be a sign that too many carbohydrates have been consumed and
thus possibly a full fat yoghurt (natural) may help to remove the
symptom. Headaches are not just because... they usually indicate
either dehydration or the over consumption of a food group. Protein
types break food down at an accelerated rate, therefore it is important
for them to avoid or seriously limit their intake of what is classed
as "caution carbohydrates" such as wholegrain bread, brown rice,
wholegrain pastas, or non-green vegetables (root vegetables such as
carrots, beets, potato, radishes, onions, yam). Other foods that are not
optimal for protein types that should also be consumed in moderation
are lettuce, green peppers, cabbages, pickles, cucumbers and tomato.

Oils/Fats
20%
EYES

Proteins
45%

Carbohydrates
35%

NO EYES

(Paul Chek - How to Eat, Move and Be Healthy 2004)

13

It is important for protein types to include protein in every meal and avoid skipping mealtimes and to ensure that they also include 'high-purine' proteins such as sardines, mussels and anchovy in their diet, as these proteins more than all the others are oxidised (converted to energy) at the proper rate for their metabolic type. For a protein type, including these in each meal greatly enhances the body's chemistry and ensures metabolism.

Like all diets, The Atkins Diet, although trashed by many, was a diet suitable for SOME but not all protein types. For carbohydrate or mixed types, this type of diet can lead to increased fat storage, and disturbed adrenal and/or thyroid function.

Some of the benefits for protein types are:

- ◆ Elimination of fatigue and lethargy
- ◆ Elimination of cravings and hyperactivity
- ◆ Maintenance of a healthy balanced appetite
- ◆ Offset degenerative disease such as cardiovascular problems, immune deficiency, blood sugar problems, digestives disorders etc

(*The Metabolic Typing Diet*, William L Wolcott)

Avoid or seriously limit foods containing the following acids:

Oxalic Acid - this naturally occurs in some foods and will interfere with the absorption of calcium, which is important for protein types. Oxalic acid is destroyed in cooking, so if the items in the following list are cooked, then they can be consumed: black tea, blackberry, beets, beet greens, chard, chocolate, cocoa, cranberries, currants (red), endive gooseberries, grapes, green peppers, plums, raspberries, rhubarb, strawberries, tomatoes. Apples, asparagus and spinach also contain oxalic acid but are exceptions.

Phytates – Phytic acid is a chemical found in bran, portions of grains and legumes. It binds with calcium, iron, magnesium, phosphorous and zinc, in the intestinal tract, subsequently preventing their absorption. This can cause mineral deficiency, allergies, and intestinal distress and bone loss. Protein types have an increased need for calcium, so excessively consuming foods with phytic acid can become problematic. The highest source of phytates are wheat, oats, soy and soy milk. The best breads for protein types are sourdough and sprouted-grain breads as their long fermentation process makes them literally phytate free. All other breads should be limited or avoided.

Vitamins that assist in optimal health

Vitamin B5 = Calcium Pantothenate

Calcium Pantothenate is a water-soluble member of the B-vitamin family. It is necessary to help with the efficient working of the adrenal gland (the gland responsible for the release of hormones in response to stress), converting food into energy, building and rebuilding cells, and stimulating growth. It helps to produce the antibodies which fight infection and counteract the negative effects from drugs and antibiotics. It also assists in the healing of most wounds.

13

Calcium Pantothenate can also help prevent fatigue and reduce mental and physical shock after major surgery or as a result of a traumatic experience. Deficiency can cause hypoglycaemia.

It can be found in: beef, kidney, liver, heart, poultry, wholegrain, bran muffins, wheatgerm, most nuts, green vegetables and yeast. It is important to note though that canned foods and preservatives, alcohol, estrogen and heat, all inhibit the absorption of this vitamin.

A POINT TO NOTE: ALCOHOL DEPLETES THE GLYCOGEN STORE IN THE LIVER CAUSING INCREASED BLOOD SUGAR LEVELS, WHICH USUALLY PROMOTES THE CRAVING OF MORE CARBOHYDRATES; INSULIN SPIKES. WHILST IT IS OPTIMAL TO HAVE LITTLE OR NO ALCOHOL, FOR POST-MENOPAUSAL WOMEN IT CAN HELP WITH ESTROGEN PRODUCTION, AS ALCOHOL CAN INCREASE THE CONVERSION OF TESTOSTERONE INTO ESTRADIOL, THUS REDUCING THEIR RISK OF CARDIOVASCULAR DISEASE WITHOUT SIGNIFICANTLY IMPAIRING BONE QUALITY OR INCREASING THEIR RISK OF ALCOHOLIC LIVER DISEASE OR BREAST CANCER.

Carbohydrate Types - Carbohydrate Types, also known as Slow Oxidisers or Sympathetics. Their appetites are not as strong as protein types and they can last longer on each meal. If you have no blood sugar regulations then you will be freer to eat high glycaemic foods, but you must not make the mistake of continually substituting all/most of your moderate or low starch carbohydrates for a plate full of these. Carbohydrate types in contrast to protein types do not convert carbohydrates as quickly into energy and thus do not do as well on dense food that takes longer to convert to 'usable' energy for the body.

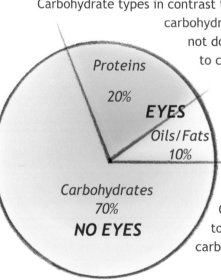

Proteins
20%
EYES
Oils/Fats
10%
Carbohydrates
70%
NO EYES

Light fish and meats, and fruit and vegetables, are far easier to break down and thus make energy more readily available. They are therefore better suited to a Carb Type.

Carbohydrate types can do well on up to 65% of the plate consisting of carbohydrates, with 25% protein and

(Paul Chek - How to Eat, Move and Be Healthy 2004)

10% fat. It is important for carbohydrate types to understand the significance of the GI index and GI load. Whilst the GI index tells you how quickly a food converts to sugar, the GI load tells you the 'impact' the food portion you have eaten will have on your system. For example, watermelon as a fruit has a high GI index, but the slice you may eat has relatively little carbohydrate so its impact on your system is relatively low (yes, it gets complicated – but if you are a diabetic it is good to understand this as you will not feel that all foods are off limits).

> " Light fish and meats, and fruit and vegetables, are far easier to break down and thus make energy more readily available. They are therefore better suited to a slow oxidiser. "

This allows you to prepare better meals, as you better understand portion size and impact. It is a big misconception that a carbohydrate or slow oxidiser can eat as much starchy food as they like because the body can handle it. If you are a slow oxidiser that does not move (exercise) this can be detrimental to your health in the long run. It is important to have a plate that is primarily green; this allows the pancreas to not have to work too hard and will also provide you with the right amount of usable energy and keep your waistline down.

A POINT TO NOTE: RAW FOOD DIETS ARE MORE COMMONPLACE TODAY BECAUSE OF THE TOTAL NUTRIENT VALUE. BUT FOR CARBOHYDRATE TYPES THE FOLLOWING FOODS EATEN RAW CAN INHIBIT THYROID FUNCTION, NEEDED FOR METABOLISM REGULATION: BROCCOLI, BRUSSEL SPROUTS, CABBAGE, CAULIFLOWER, KALE, MUSTARD, RUTABAGA AND WATERCRESS.

It is therefore advisable to supplement your diet with kelp, as this gives the body extra iodine, the absorption of which is blocked because of the presence of goitrogen, a substance that can cause thyroid dysfunction. (*The Metabolic Typing® Diet* by William L Wolcott)

13

Mixed Type - Mixed Type, also known as mixed oxidisers or balanced autonomic dominants, are somewhere in-between protein and carbohydrate types. Mixed types fall into two categories that are dependent on their characteristics including strengths/weaknesses, energy levels, strength of appetite and the way they react to the foods they eat:

Oils/Fats
10%

EYES

Proteins
40%

Carbohydrat
50%
NO EYES

◆ **Type A** – means that most of the characteristics do not display either dominance towards protein or carbohydrate type. This type is truly 'neutral', with a tendency to have an average appetite, hungry usually only at mealtimes.

◆ **Type R** – means that there is a tendency to have relative measures/strong traits of both protein and carbohydrate dominance as opposed to neutral, with a tendency to sometimes feel ravenous (protein type trait) and then not feel hungry and even skip meals (carbohydrate type trait).

Mixed types must ensure that they use both food charts effectively to ensure optimal health, trim waistlines and enhanced wellbeing. As they are neither fast nor slow oxidisers it is important for them to mix the types of proteins and fats they consume daily, eating the ideal foods for both protein and carbohydrate types to ensure their bodies function efficiently. Mixed oxidisers generally have an average appetite and little problem in trying to control their weight, but they do tend to be prone to fatigue, anxiety and nervousness (*The Metabolic Typing® Diet* by William L Wolcott).

The two main pathways that affect every cell in our bodies are known as the sympathetic and parasympathetic pathways. These two pathways are responsible for our fright/flight responses and the rest/restoration of our bodies. The sympathetic pathways are responsible for shutting down the digestive system and preparing the body for the stresses it may face. Pupil dilation, increased heart rate, contraction of the lungs, activation of sweat gland secretion, digestive tract inhibition (peristalsis; pushing waste towards the anal canal for elimination) and even the promotion of ejaculation from the penis, are all examples of sympathetic pathways dominance.

> 66 *Our body's systems must be balanced, neither too acidic nor too alkaline. Chemotherapy, free radical damage, stress etcetera, can all leave the system very unbalanced and in a weakened position* 99

Parasympathetic dominance is responsible for the rest of the body's functions and digestion when the body is at rest. It is also responsible for sexual arousal, salivation, tears, urination and defecation, in opposition to the sympathetic pathway.

These two systems alone play massive roles in sexual arousal, activity, ejaculation and reproduction, so once again it is necessary to understand their influence on pelvic floor conditioning and sexual function. The dominance of these two systems exists across all Metabolic Types® and is usually only realised as the diet is fine-tuned or by a thorough metabolic assessment that usually takes a couple of weeks.

13

Our body's systems must be balanced, neither too acidic nor too alkaline. Chemotherapy, free radical damage, stress etcetera, can all leave the system very unbalanced and in a weakened position, so it is imperative to optimal health that you know which foods and/or natural organic food supplements will help to bring this to pass. It is also crucial that you understand the significance of the quality of the water that you drink.

Water with a pH of 7.2 or above is naturally more alkaline and will supply more oxygen to the body's systems and help to neutralise it. For cancer patients this is imperative, but for optimal health it is also vital. My sister recently pointed out that Evian spelt naïve backwards; and you are naïve if you do not recognise that Evian is good for you. Evian should be the minimum standard of your water quality; Panna, the 'still sister' of San Pellegrino has a pH of 8.2, making it an even better choice in terms of alkalinity.

We also need to include turmeric, cinnamon and fenugreek into our diet, as standard, as well as wheatgrass by Pure-XP, which has neutralising (alkalising) properties (please note that this is not the case for some fast oxidisers). You should also consume fruit such as papaya and vegetables like broccoli and slightly cooked tomatoes, for their levels of lycopene, which is said to have good cancer halting benefits. Weight Watchers make billions not from getting results but from the program that weighs you. Weight Watchers use some of the most amazing health clubs, housing all of the facilities that can optimise health, weight and wellbeing. Yet women walk in, get weighed and then walk straight back out, without using any of these facilities; how does that ensure education, postural and structural wellbeing and not just pounds lost?

Our bodies require that we drink at least half our body weight in fluid ounces daily. The calculation is bodyweight x 0.0333. In kindness to you I have worked out the amounts needed from 9st – 12st, just to give you a real idea of what you should be drinking. I have done it averaging, but the sum is there for you should you need it:

Weight:	Water Intake:
9st – 9st 4lbs	1.9ltrs – 1.97ltrs
9st 5lbs – 9st 9lbs	1.98 – 2.04ltrs
9st 10lbs – 10st	2.05 – 2.12ltrs
10st 1lbs – 10st 5lbs	2.13 – 2.19ltrs
10st 6lbs – 10st 10lbs	2.20 – 2.27ltrs
10st 11lbs – 11st	2.29 – 2.33ltrs
11st 1lb – 11st 5lbs	2.35 – 2.40lts
11st 6lbs – 11st 10lbs	2.42 – 2.48lts
11st 11lbs – 12st	2.49 – 2.54lts

A POINT TO NOTE: YOUR BODY WILL SACRIFICE YOUR REPAIR HORMONES AND SEX HORMONES TO MAKE WAY FOR YOUR STRESS HORMONES. THIS IS A CRUCIAL POINT FOR THOSE TRYING TO HAVE A FAMILY OR FOR INDIVIDUALS TRYING TO LOSE WEIGHT.

Summary

In summary no one diet plan works for EVERYBODY! Our body's reaction to food: combination, portions, times, etc and the systems which dominants within each individual, is an education in itself. It means that we need to pay more attention to what, when and how we eat if we want to truly optimise our health, and our environmental, mental emotional and spiritual factors play an ongoing part.

13

THE EXERCISES:
Strengthening the Pelvic Floor Muscles

WELL we have made it to this section where we will be putting the information into action. For the most effective results it would be advisable to consider having a full plumb line postural assessment at some point in the future, as this allows you to know just how balanced you really are from head to foot. If you want the poor man's answer immediately – get someone to take four pictures of you in just your bra and knickers. One from behind, one in front and it is very important you take two side on, one looking left and one looking right! You will then be able to see for yourself the position of your feet, knees, hips, shoulders and head. Whilst you can see the curves of the shoulders and lower back, you cannot measure them and that is crucial. I have not told you what we look for when doing a postural assessment, but I bet when you relax into your normal stance and then see the pictures you will be surprised at how you actually stand!

> " Great posture and a fully functional system is not only very sexy, it is damn empowering and that is what allows a woman to glide gracefully and graciously. "

Balanced training is NOT doing the same exercise in equal numbers on the right and left, but rather finding out what is short and tight vs. what is weak and lengthened, and then redressing. Once the body is balanced then equal work, stretch, reps etcetera can be carried out.

Pelvic Floor Secrets does not offer a service that just looks at one area, i.e. the vagina; it looks at the whole body, as the position of the feet, knees, hips, head, the shape of the butt and the curvature of the spine all play a massive part in pelvic floor function. I have always been a head to toe girl; I never believe in just focusing on one part to look good.

Great posture and a fully functional system is not only very sexy, it is damn empowering and that is what allows a woman to glide gracefully and graciously.

We are, as I have mentioned before, a kinetic chain, with most of our structural issues being more visible at the top. Look at the totem pole right and see that the further up the chain you go, the more stress is placed lower down, with our pelvic floor being right at the line that joins the upper and lower body together. If the upper part is out of kilter, it must impact the lower part and thus both parts impact the pelvic floor.

The beauty of breathing

In order to master pelvic floor and lower abdominal training you first need to master the art of diaphragmatic breathing and I do mean the art of breathing, because many of us have developed what I call man at the bar breath, where we pull everything inwards in the hope to make the torso appear leaner. The problem with this kind

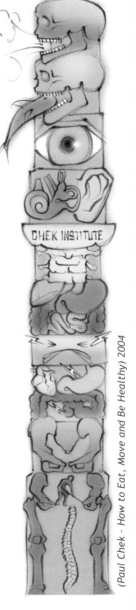

(Paul Chek - How to Eat, Move and Be Healthy) 2004

> *When you optimise your breathing your ability to fully grip your partner is maximised, and the better you grip the more likely you are to have a vaginal orgasm, which is far more powerful and explosive than a clitoral orgasm without a doubt.*

of breathing, also known as inverted breathing, is that it restricts the airways, not allowing oxygen to get all the way to our toes, causing us to recruit the wrong muscles, thereby not giving them the workout they need which can also lead to postural imbalances. It also means that you do not fully oxygenate your pelvic floor, which needs blood flow for optimal efficiency, especially if we are hoping to have amazing orgasms.

When you optimise your breathing your ability to fully grip your partner is maximised, and the better you grip the more likely you are to have a vaginal orgasm, which is far more powerful and explosive than a clitoral orgasm without a doubt.

Oxygen, which is nutrition for your body, is crucial to the health and function of the brain, the heart, lungs, all the internal organs, every single cell in the body and your pelvic floor. Everything within the body requires an ongoing 'optimal' supply of oxygen in order to continue to function at 100%. Many do not realise the importance of optimal oxygen flow for good pelvic floor health; we focus on specific exercises to improve aesthetics without realising that optimising the flow of oxygen to the relative muscle, significantly improves its energy output, function and tone.

Diaphragmatic Breath Standing No.1

◆ Stand in front of a mirror and take a deep breathe in through the nose. What do you see? If your chest and shoulders elevate, this is what is known as inverted breathing (restricted within the ribcage). If inhaled correctly, the tummy should expand without the shoulders or chest elevating. Exhale through

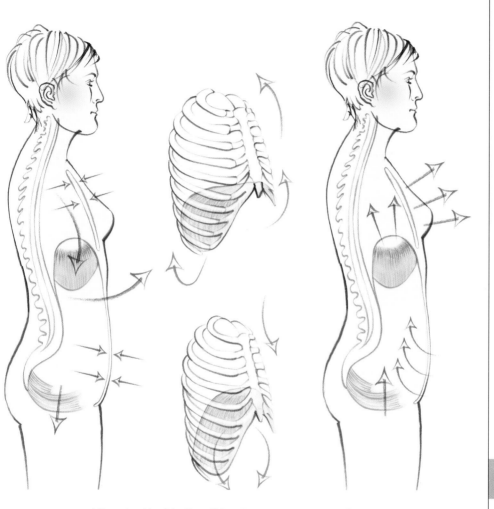

pursed lips (as if whistling/blowing a trumpet) and empty/
shrink the tummy. As you exhale, focus on what happens to your
vagina (or testes) and abdomen. You should feel a slight pulling
in and up through the vagina (or testes) and the belly button
should begin to retract. It is not an action that requires you to
focus or physically pull the belly button as such, but rather an

14

automatic kinetic reaction because of elevation within the pelvic floor. The two work on the same fire wire and so as one moves so too should the other, in complete synchronisation.

When you take a deep breath in through the nose, firstly, it sounds deep. The shoulders and chest should not move, but rather the tummy should expand, as the oxygen comes into it. Think of putting air into a balloon/ball, expanding as the air goes in. As the lungs expand and elevate, the respiratory diaphragm drops and the viscera - our internal organs and pelvic diaphragm drop also putting a little more pressure on our pelvic organs. You should feel a little downward pressure on your pelvic floor; a great way to identify it. And as you breathe out, both the pelvic and respiratory diaphragm move back into place, picking everything up. You should then feel an upward motion between the vagina or penis, and the anus, the perineum. This is the pelvic floor being "picked up." This is sensory programming no.1, where breathing is everything.

A POINT TO NOTE: NOT EVERYONE CAN IDENTIFY THEIR PELVIC FLOOR OR INDEED MASTER THE DIAPHRAGMATIC BREATHING IN THE STANDING POSITION. THEREFORE THIS EXERCISE CAN BE REPEATED EITHER ON ALL FOURS (SEE DIAGRAMS ON PAGE 199 OR LYING ON YOUR BACK, SEE PAGE 203) ONCE YOU FIND THE POSITION THAT BEST SUITS YOU, THIS IS YOUR INITIAL POSITION OF STRENGTH. MASTER IT FIRST, BUT, ALWAYS ENDEAVOUR TO MASTER ALL THREE AS THESE ARE ALL FUNCTIONAL POSITIONS.

Diaphragmatic Breath Standing No.2
Once you can identify the breath, you need to now advance it for optimal pelvic floor function.

◆ Take a deep breath in and hold it. As you breathe in, your vagina feels as if it is opening up and something is moving down as the lips part (The testicles should descend away from the body). Whilst holding your breath, try and draw the vaginal lips together as if closing a zip and then elevate the floor upwards towards the belly button (as if zipping up) and exhale (Men, imagine you are taking the testicles from the ground floor to the penthouse). As you exhale hold the elevation that should actually feel as though it has intensified. Your belly button will naturally begin to draw towards the spine, activation from the floor upwards.

> " Ladies, it is important to note that the sensations felt are activated within the vaginal canal as opposed to feeling as if you are stopping wind. It is a gentle feeling but one that you can identify over time and come to realise it is a front to back feeling, crucial for heightened sexual pleasure. "

Ladies, it is important to note that the sensations felt are activated within the vaginal canal as opposed to feeling as if you are stopping wind. It is a gentle feeling but one that you can identify over time and come to realise it is a front to back feeling, crucial for heightened sexual pleasure.

This way of activating the pelvic floor is heightened sensory programming that ensures identification right at the root. It will be the way in which you use your core for all activity; a functional contraction of the pelvic floor and lower abdominals that will maximise support, continence and protection for the lower back.

14

Master this technique first then consider load afterwards! Allow yourself 10-20 minutes per workout three times per week minimum, for optimal results. You do not need to do the 20 minutes in one hit, but can split it

> Sarah and Nicci both suffered with vaginisimus for years in their early twenties, and found intimate relationships very hard. By mastering their diaphragmatic breathing they have found that it has significantly reduced the condition, allowing the vagina to relax, making lovemaking an exciting prospect.

throughout the day. Most of us have what is known as faulty breathing habits and it is our body's position of strength or engram (a position that is recognised by the brain automatically). To undo a faulty engram can take between 3-5,000 reps, hence the workout to redress the way we breathe.

If you are not sure how the two work in unison, then try sticking your thumb in the roof of your mouth and sucking hard on it. You should feel the contraction or pulling up within the vagina or testes and a subsequent co-contraction through the belly button. This is a very visible sign that the two work on the same neurological loop, with the belly button naturally beginning a 'retreat' from front to back, just as nature designed. Many of us only struggle to feel it, simply because we have not learnt how to switch on the sensory pathway effectively.

A POINT TO NOTE: THERE ARE A NUMBER OF EXERCISES THAT CAN FOLLOW ON FROM HERE THAT ARE AMAZING NOT ONLY FOR THE PELVIC FLOOR BUT ALSO FOR THE LOWER ABDOMINALS, UPPER BACK, SHOULDERS, TRICEPS AND MORE IMPORTANTLY POSTURAL ALIGNMENT. HORSE STANCE IN MANY PLANES IS A GREAT EXERCISE AND BOOKS LIKE PAUL CHEK'S *HOW TO EAT, MOVE AND BE HEALTHY* OR LEIGH BRANDON'S *ANATOMY SERIES*, ALLOW YOU TO INCORPORATE THE PELVIC FLOOR ON THE GO. WE PROGRESS YOUR CONDITIONING PROGRAM IN THIS WAY, ACCORDING TO THE PROGRAM CHOSEN AND THE RESULTS OF YOUR POSTURAL, VAGINAL AND PHYSICAL ASSESSMENT.

Seated Pelvic Floor

You can do this exercise in two ways, firstly identifying the pelvic floor by sitting on the edge of a chair and then progressing to sitting cross-legged on the floor:

◆ Sit on a chair with your knees slightly apart and imagine you are trying to stop yourself from passing wind. Without moving your buttocks or your legs, focus and try to squeeze the muscle just above the entrance of your anus. You should feel a gentle movement in the muscle.

◆ Now I want you to focus on the vagina and imagine you are trying to stop yourself from urinating. You should find that you have to squeeze a different part of the pelvic floor, within the vagina (or testes) itself. Again the buttocks and legs should stay still. You can feel the buttocks move if you pull from the wrong place. It is the muscles from the front that I want you to strengthen! If you are unsure of these muscles then use what we call 'poor man's biofeedback', and place a couple of fingers inside the vagina (or rest your middle finger on the testes). Your vagina should gently close against them when you do this identifying exercise (or your testes begin to move upward).

Now you are ready to do pelvic floor exercises, which you should endeavour to do daily at first. Our sensory pathways are unique to us; some of us can identify the exercise better on all fours, others find it easier sitting, and others find it easier lying on their backs. None of them are wrong and over time all of them are worth mastering. I usually get my clients to try all three positions and then master the one they feel gives them the best feedback. Once they have mastered one, they can move on and master the others. We must be able to activate

14

" *It is important for you to exercise the correct muscles within the vaginal canal, as mentioned earlier.* "

our pelvic floor in all planes in order to be able to use it functionally: at work, at home, carrying our children, intimately and in all activities. Pelvic floor on the go must be your ultimate goal.

It takes time, practice and discipline to become good at any exercise, but remember that these exercises offer support, protection, aesthetics (especially lower abdominals and buttocks), continence, empowerment, confidence and increased sexual satisfaction. Many people ask, "How long before I experience any results?" and the answer really is, "How long is a piece of string?" Within as little as six weeks you can begin to 'feel' a significant improvement provided you do the exercise religiously. If your sensory pathways are awake then results will be experienced earlier still.

At my clinic in Central London, I offer a sensory service where you can see from the feedback on the computer just how awake your pelvic floor is and this then gives your starting point. We also use this in the programs to chart progress over the six weeks. It is an empowering position to be in, to be able to see the improvement visually on a chart, week by week. www.pelvicfloorsecrets.com

Four-point Tummy Vacuum 1

◆ Get onto the floor on all fours, with hands under the shoulders and knees under the hips. Keep your head parallel to the floor and shoulders drawn away from the ears, down towards the hips. Try and rotate the pelvic area by rolling the hips forwards and backwards without moving the upper body. Watch out for rounding of the upper body and elevation of the shoulders towards the ears. It is important to try and maintain

Four-point Tummy Vacuum

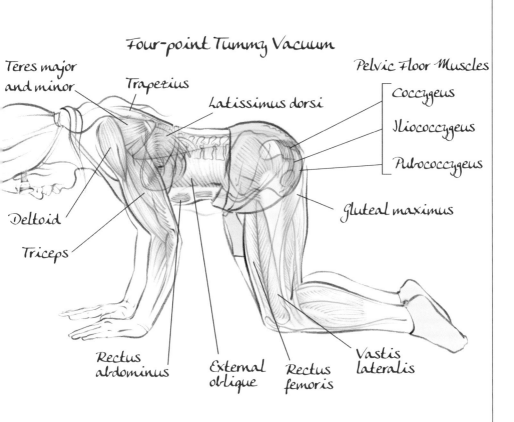

Teres major and minor

Trapezius

Latissimus dorsi

Pelvic Floor Muscles

Coccygeus

Iliococcygeus

Pubococcygeus

Gluteal maximus

Deltoid

Triceps

Rectus abdominus

External oblique

Rectus femoris

Vastis lateralis

good posture. Rotation of the hips; disassociation of the upper and lower body is good for the pelvic floor and transfers to intimacy.

Inhale and rotate the pelvis backwards (tipping your bottom up towards the ceiling), creating a dip in the lower back without moving the mid back. Exhale through pursed lips and roll the bottom under. You should feel your pelvic floor elevating with breath. Hold for five seconds and as you inhale to repeat, release your pelvic floor (you should have that feeling of your vagina opening as mentioned above).

14

It is important for you to exercise the correct muscles within the vaginal canal, as mentioned earlier.

Identifying the muscles is the key to optimal pelvic floor training and many times it is the recruitment of the dominant outer muscles that fire before the deep inner muscles really get the chance to work, which is why the identification and sense of warmth is a true indicator that you are working the correct muscles.

A great way to gauge the condition of your pelvic floor is with a laugh or a cough using what is known as a 'poor man's biofeedback.' Make yourself laugh or cough and focus on what happens within the vagina (or testes) and the lower abdominals. If the pelvic floor is conditioned then you should feel a nice little tug within the canal and the belly button should retract slightly. Note that as you laugh or cough, your buttocks do not make a significant contraction as they do if you recruit from the back to front. The stronger the feeling, the more conditioned the floor may be and will then require a strength program. The weaker the contraction, the more work is needed to awaken the sensory pathways first, before the strengthening phase can begin. Sorry, you have to awaken that floor before you can strengthen it.

Four Point Tummy Vacuum 2

This exercise now includes pelvic floor awakening, advancing the exercise by adding correct pelvic floor elevation.

◆ Keeping the same postural position as four point 1, inhale and feel the pelvic floor 'falling'/opening into the vagina as the lips part. Whilst holding your breath, close the lips and focus on elevating up toward the belly button. Exhale through pursed lips and feel the elevation increase and the contraction intensify. Focus inside the vagina as opposed to the perineum and imagine the lips are the sides of a zip. Draw them together and then begin to pull the zip up, pulling your pelvic floor towards your belly button.

Hold the elevation for three seconds initially, and then release it as you inhale again and 'allow the zip to undo.' Three seconds is a long time to 'hold' the floor and trying to hold for longer, initially, tends to recruit other bigger muscles which is when the faulty patterns begin. Start with 10 reps, with a three second hold, resting for 45 seconds and repeating three times = 30 holds. Try and work up to doing six sets of 10 x three second holds, so that the 'time under tension' allows the muscles to adapt and condition.

> 66 *Sucking the thumb, laughter, coughing and so on should activate a movement not just from downstairs but from behind the belly button.* 99

It is important to remember also that you have fast and slow twitch fibres within the pelvic floor and whilst most of the fibres are slow twitch you do need to improve the fast twitch also because they are put under pressure when you begin many activities including intimacy.

Once you have adequately mastered switching these muscles on and can bring about a real warm and deep abdominal workout, try and include a set where there is no time held, but rather you 'zip' and 'unzip' rhythmically so that this strength can be transferred into the bedroom, the exercise class and whenever you are on the go.

14

When you have comfortably mastered your six sets of ten reps with a three second hold, increase the 'holding time' by two seconds and decrease the sets by one e.g.: 5 sets of 10 reps with a 5 second hold. Continue to increase the seconds to 7 and 10 second holds, whilst decreasing to 4 and 3 sets respectively.

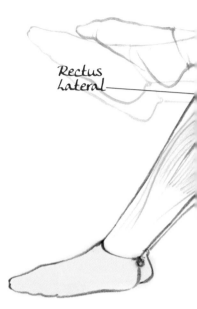

Rectus Lateral

The same exercise can now be repeated either sitting with your legs crossed or lying on your back with your knees bent. The breathing is exactly the same.

A POINT TO NOTE: I WILL ALWAYS TEACH PELVIC FLOOR EXERCISES IN CONJUNCTION WITH BREATHING BECAUSE THAT IS THE WAY THE BODY IS WIRED AND AS DISCUSSED EARLIER THE BODY IS A KINETIC CHAIN. AS MENTIONED, SUCKING THE THUMB, LAUGHTER, COUGHING AND SO ON SHOULD ACTIVATE A MOVEMENT NOT JUST FROM DOWNSTAIRS BUT FROM BEHIND THE BELLY BUTTON.

It is important though when you do these exercises not to pull from the trunk first, but instead to pull from the vagina and then feel the movement 'travel' up towards the belly button.

Lower Abdominal One (LA1)

To work the lower abdominals effectively you will need to invest in a blood pressure cuff. This will allow you to visually identify how stable your trunk is. You can order the cuff from my website or find a local pharmacy that should sell them. If you do not have one for now then use your hand as a point of reference and try to maintain the same pressure.

Lower Abdominal One

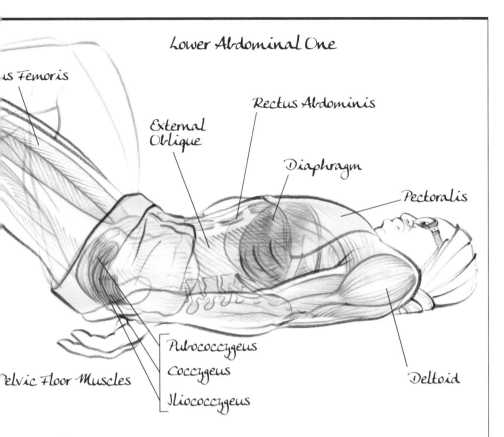

us Femoris

External Oblique

Rectus Abdominis

Diaphragm

Pectoralis

Pelvic Floor Muscles

Pubococcygeus

Coccygeus

Iliococcygeus

Deltoid

◆ Lie on your back with knees bent and place the cuff in the lower back in line with your belly button. Pump the cuff until the needle is at 40mm/hg, acting as the natural curve in the lower back. Inhale and, as you exhale, draw the pelvic floor, via the vagina or testes, toward the belly button and then tip the pelvis back towards your face so that your lower back is pushed against the cuff and the needle rises to 70mm/hg.

The objective is to keep the needle as still as possible at 70mm/hg +/- 5mm/hg whilst breathing diaphragmatically. Breathe in and as you exhale begin to pull the pelvic floor up towards the belly button. Hold for three seconds and then release it as you inhale again. The needle should be as still as possible +/- 5mm/hg. If you do not have a cuff, you can use your hands, fingertips touching, maintaining a constant pressure on your hand. Repeat for one minute, rest for thirty seconds and start again. Complete three sets of one minute breathing.

Lower Abdominal Two (LA2)

Once you have mastered lower abdominal one, and are confident that you can keep the needle stable, progress onto this exercise. It is encouraging to want to move forward, but make sure you have mastered the base or foundation exercises first to ensure the recruitment will always come from the right place. There are many muscles around the pelvic floor that will 'take over', usually because they have been recruited falsely from the start so stay patient as you empower yourself.

◆ Lie on your back with your knees bent as in LA1 and place the blood pressure cuff (or your hand) behind the belly button in the small of the back. Pump the cuff until the needle is at 40mm/hg. Inhale, and as you exhale draw the pelvic floor, via the vagina or testes, toward the belly button, then tip the pelvis back towards your face so that your lower back is pushed against the cuff and the needle rises to 70mm/hg.

Take a diaphragmatic breath in and whilst holding that breath engage the pelvic floor, by closing the vaginal lips and 'zipping' up (or lifting the testes) so that you not only feel it elevate but you also feel the belly button pulling back in concert. Moving from the hip, lift one leg from the floor, to a 90 degree angle at the hip. Hold for two seconds and then exhale and lower. Alternate and repeat 10 times each side. Again the needle should be as still as possible at +/- 5mm/hg.

If you find it too hard to keep still you are not ready for this exercise yet and need to improve the stability of your breathing. Regress the exercise to lifting the heel off the floor first, moving to just lifting the foot, before finally pulling the leg higher.

Ultimately you would want to progress this exercise to standing, placing the blood pressure cuff against a column. This is a great way of showing that the pelvic floor is functional and can work in our everyday life.

Meet your Body

It is important to understand posture and its effects on pelvic floor function so we now look at the way we stand. In Noah Karresch's book, Meet your Body, he has a six-point foot position which helps to activate the proprioception in our feet. It is very enlightening and also hard for many. The tingles, numbness and/or tightness you feel are all those muscles in the feet that are shut down by our footwear. Yes, it is what we wear that can mess up how we move and function.

◆ Stand with your feet just outside of hip width, with feet facing forward. Come onto your big and little toes and whilst maintaining the weight evenly between these two points, roll back onto the balls of the feet behind the toes and then make contact with the heels along these two lines. You have six points of contact with the ground, try and keep them even. For those of us (including me) whose feet pronate, this is very hard. Next look down at your knees and if they are not over the second toe, rotate them laterally through sense, not physically.

14

These two positions alone should be giving you some feedback. The lateral rotation of the knee 'switches on' the inner thighs, the hips and buttocks, and the new feelings go right up into the private area; as if by magic. Now place a hand just above the pubic bone and in the small

> 66 *The primary role of the buttocks is to extend the hip, support the pelvic floor and keep the knees and feet in a neutral alignment to the trunk so the feet do not roll in on themselves, creating problems like flat feet* 99

of the back, and rotate your pelvis a fraction until you feel a little pull along the pubic line, then lift the chest, without moving the set pelvis, and draw your head back as if you are being double chinned; I bet your body is talking big time.

For most of us women, the conversation our body has with us, about our ankles, under our feet, through our butts, inside our thighs, and more importantly inside our vagina, gives a clear indication of the kinetic chain that we are and the reason why we cannot focus on just one place. Paul Chek's totem pole is truly an eye opener and shows just how we load ourselves and what systems are impacted.

With that in mind let's look at the buttocks, in particular the medial part, and see what exactly is going on.

The primary role of the buttocks is to extend the hip, support the pelvic floor and keep the knees and feet in a neutral alignment to the trunk so the feet do not roll in on themselves, creating problems like flat feet, which then cause the knees to start to play music by becoming knocked/rolling and then shutting down the muscles of the hips and buttocks which can lead to an inefficient pelvic floor.

The 'clam' exercise

This is a good isolator of the medial buttock's muscles, which play an important part in the stability of pelvic floor muscles. The medial buttock abducts and externally rotates the hip, and is a lateral stabiliser of the pelvis, stopping the hips from collapsing in onto the pelvic girdle;

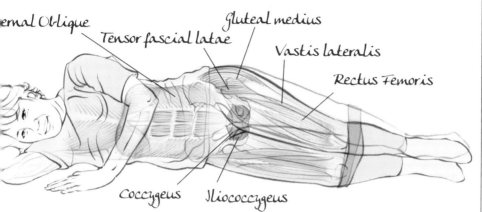

The clam exercise

ernal Oblique
Tensor fascial latae
Gluteal medius
Vastis lateralis
Rectus Femoris
Coccygeus
Iliococcygeus

◆ Lie on your right side with your hips flexed to 30 degrees and the knees and feet bent and lying together on top of each other. The objective is to open the top knee without moving either the heels or more importantly the pelvis. It is a way of measuring isolation and correct recruitment of the muscle, not using the TFL, tensor fascia latae, which is also a hip abductor muscle and serves to help steady the pelvis on the head of the femur (top of the hip). As you begin to open the knees, you should not move very far but you should feel tension in the middle of the hip (butt). You can hold this position and use your fingers to palpate the muscle and make sure it switches on. Try and hold the tension for up to 3 minutes, this can be done as 6 reps each being held for 30 seconds, palpating intermittently. Your butt should feel alive, a necessary requirement for optimal pelvic floor conditioning. You can isolate this exercise further by adding a resistance band around the knees. Do not "over force" the opening, instead "work with" the resistance without compromising posture.

14

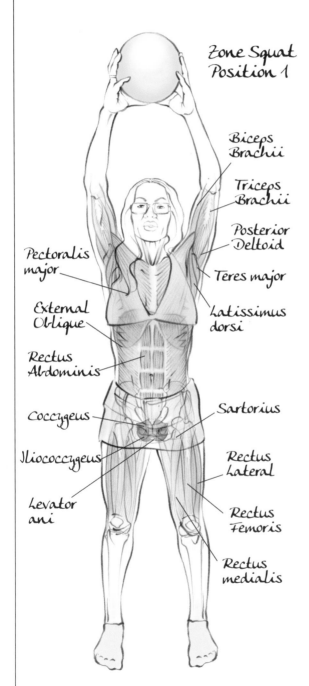

Zone Squat
Position 1

Biceps
Brachii

Triceps
Brachii

Posterior
Deltoid

Teres major

Latissimus
dorsi

Pectoralis
major

External
Oblique

Rectus
Abdominis

Coccygeus

Iliococcygeus

Levator
ani

Sartorius

Rectus
Lateral

Rectus
Femoris

Rectus
medialis

Zone Squat

The zone squat is a great exercise, not only for optimising the airways, but also as a great way to use the pelvic floor in a functional exercise. It is also a good way to improve the squat pattern that so many people tend to struggle with. This is a synchronised exercise that requires a good amount of practice and it is important that this exercise is led by the breathing and synchronised accordingly:

◆ Stand with feet hip width apart and raise your arms up above your head. Think of your body as a sheet of paper that will fold from the middle first and then fold at the knees. Take a diaphragmatic breath in and whilst holding that for a second, draw the vaginal lips together and 'zip up' towards the bellybutton. Try keeping your pelvic floor elevated

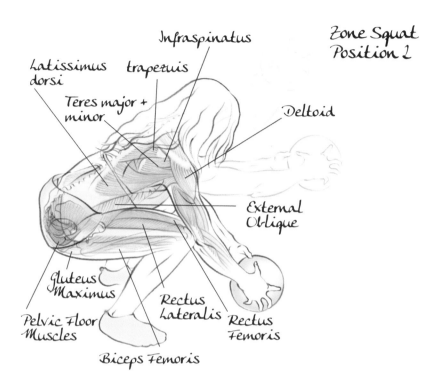

Zone Squat
Position 2

Infraspinatus

Latissimus dorsi

trapezuis

Teres major + minor

Deltoid

External Oblique

Gluteus Maximus

Pelvic Floor Muscles

Rectus Lateralis

Rectus Femoris

Biceps Femoris

as you exhale and begin to 'fold' at the hips, descending towards the floor. Your bottom should end up below your knees and your hands should come down last. Hold for one second and release your pelvic floor, then lift your arms over your head, as if you are giving your hands to someone to help you up. Inhale as you begin to stand, letting the arms lead and unfold the body. Repeat without breaking the breathing.

◆ Start with 8-12 reps, 3 sets with 60 seconds, and rest in-between. Make sure your feet remain flat throughout; if the heels begin to lift, take the feet further apart.

14

This exercise is good for improving the strength of the buttocks, thighs, lower back and pelvic floor in a functional capacity, as well as optimising oxygen and energy flow around the body.

Activating the medial buttocks can also be done by standing up against a wall:

◆ Stand sideways next to a wall and place the forearm on it. Lift the knee closest to the wall and place the thigh against it at a 90 degree angle. Relax the arm onto the thigh and use the opposite hand to gently tap along the outside of the cheek on the standing leg. Tap continuously for 15 seconds and relax. Repeat six times on each side.

Back Lunge

The back lunge is a great practical and functional exercise that not only tests pelvic floor strength and stability but also uses it in conjunction with gait, the buttocks and lower limbs. My "Nice Legs, Good Butt" chant we used to use in class coupled with a functional pelvic floor is a must.

◆ Stand with feet hip width apart and toes pointing forward. Take a diaphragmatic breath, as described in exercise one, and elevate your pelvic floor whilst holding. Step back with your right leg remaining at hip width and curl the toes as the foot lands. Allow the hips to drop to create a 90/90 at both knees. Hold for 2 seconds and then pushing through the front foot, exhale and extend up, bringing the back foot in line with the front. Repeat on the same side for 8 reps then change sides.

Try this for 14 days before increasing the reps and sets to 2-3 sets. You can over time increase the intensity by adding weight to your hands and you can also vary the distance the feet are apart.

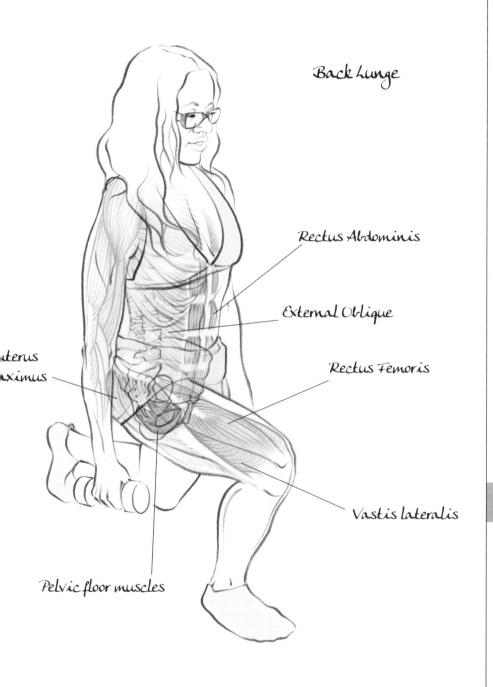

Back Lunge

Rectus Abdominis

External Oblique

Rectus Femoris

...terus
...ximus

Vastis lateralis

Pelvic floor muscles

14

Squats and lunges are the two most important functional exercises to master as they are used in everyday movements; sitting, going to the toilet, picking up the children's toys as you walk past etcetera.

There are many other exercises that can be done once these are mastered, but it would be unprofessional to offer a variety of advanced exercises without qualifying clients. The exercises above will greatly improve the efficiency and function of your pelvic floor (provided all the muscles within the pelvic basin are 'active') and offset dysfunction if you make them a part of your lifestyle choice. To increase the tone in the area, you need to invest in specific strengthening aids and the Gyneflex™ is the best on the market. It is the 'Thigh Master' for the vagina. Effective and easy to use:

Gyneflex™

The Gyneflex™ is a female's must-have accessory! It is a revolutionary vaginal muscle "strength training system" designed and patented in 2000 by gynaecologist Dr Daniel Stein FACOG and Suzanne Sloan. It is the only

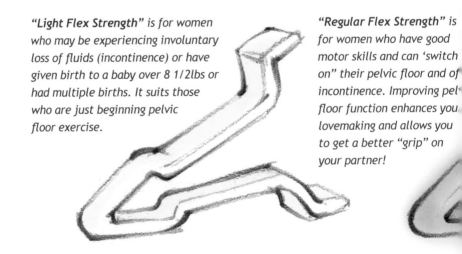

"Light Flex Strength" is for women who may be experiencing involuntary loss of fluids (incontinence) or have given birth to a baby over 8 1/2lbs or had multiple births. It suits those who are just beginning pelvic floor exercise.

"Regular Flex Strength" is for women who have good motor skills and can 'switch on" their pelvic floor and of incontinence. Improving pel floor function enhances you lovemaking and allows you to get a better "grip" on your partner!

product of its kind that is anatomically correct in its design product that truly strengthens the pelvic floor and is approved by the Federal Drugs Authority (FDA). Unlike other vaginal conditioning systems on the market, the Gyneflex™ is a single molded unit, with no moving parts or springs, which makes it more comfortable and easy to use and aesthetically friendly.

Available in five strengths plus an initial "trainer" the Gyneflex™ helps to plump up the vaginal walls and condition the pelvic floor. The end result of having these "specific weights" for your vagina is firm more conditioned muscles of the vaginal canal and pelvic floor. This 'plumped up' effect from the muscles that now have tone and body means that the 'space' between the sidewalls is narrowed, as toned muscles do not lie flat. This allows for a better 'grip' and enhanced orgasms = 'better sex' but it also means that the instance of a prolapsed pelvic organ is minimised and helps to prevent an organ from descending into the vaginal canal, because of the tautness created. Gyneflex™ is a very clever tool. The first strength, known as the 'trainer', has no resistance whatsoever. It is designed to ensure that the recruitment of the pelvic floor is correct. Many women

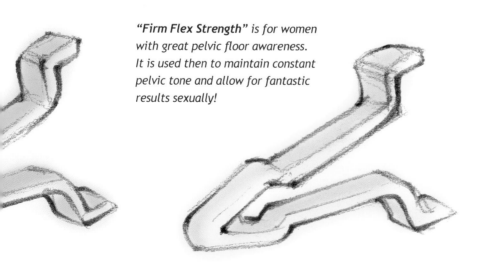

"Firm Flex Strength" is for women with great pelvic floor awareness. It is used then to maintain constant pelvic tone and allow for fantastic results sexually!

14

> **"** *The truth is the contraction from inside the vaginal wall should not cause you to have to do acrobatics or make you feel like you are desperately stopping yourself from passing wind.* **"**

do not want to believe they have no strength down there, so they will use their bottoms, inner thighs, outer abdominals, and/or hold their breath, whatever gives the impression that they can move the thing. The truth is the contraction from inside the vaginal wall should not cause you to have to do acrobatics or make you feel like you are desperately stopping yourself from passing wind. The contraction within the vagina is synchronised with a gentle tensioning that is identified from within immediately (look at the exercise section again to identify the correct muscle). I suggest that you place the soles of your feet together and allow your knees to turn out when you first start to use your Gyneflex™. This way, it is virtually impossible to recruit the buttocks or inner thighs. By placing the soles of your feet in this position you help to isolate the vagina and thus are better able to ensure correct recruitment.

Also it is good to place the palm of the hand under the low back to create the natural curve in the lower back. You can either leave the hand there or remove it, but keep this curve as it helps to further isolate the vaginal muscles/pelvic floor and ensure that there is no 'outside assistance.' Use the trainer for at least 21 days and develop the motor engram or position of strength before you go on to start using the first strength. It is not a race and in order to ensure optimal strength and conditioning it is worth working through all the strengths effectively. Once you can close the sides together and maintain the contractions for a minimum of 10 seconds for 21 consecutive days, you are ready for the next progression. Trust me, it is worth the investment, not just for sexual pleasure and amazing orgasms, but also for enhanced support of the whole pelvic floor and thus the maintenance of the organs in their correct position as you remain *confidently continent!*

A POINT TO NOTE: THE GYNEFLEX™ AS WITH STANDARD RESISTANCE TRAINING REQUIRES THE MASTERING OF THE TECHNIQUE FIRST AND THE LOAD APPLIED AFTERWARDS. JUST AS YOU LEARN THE WAY YOUR JOB WORKS BEFORE YOU LOOK FOR ELEVATION AND PROMOTION, YOU CANNOT EXPECT PROMOTION (GREAT SEX) WITHOUT PUTTING THE WORK IN FIRST.

When women come to my clinic for help to improve their pelvic platform and increase the sensation felt during penetration, many say that they only have feeling at the entrance to the vagina and not along the canal. Many of these women have spent years of doing pelvic floor exercises in part.

Vaginal strengtheners are necessary to improve and maintain tone but surprisingly women look at them with distain and many will not entertain the idea. I find this fascinating because many women today have vaginal toys for stimulation again at the tip, but not along the canal. Gyneflex™ and I are best friends. All fully functioning muscles contract and relax and the Gyenflex™ is perfect for this. The six strengths are like the dumbbells for your vagina. As your strength increases so too can the resistance. As it inserts into the vaginal canal it contours the vaginal walls that you need to use to close it, not the external part of the vagina. This promotes great co-ordination for lovemaking and is a transferable skill. No matter what other sexual aids you have, you must have and use a Gyneflex™.

When it comes to gripping your partner, co-ordination is the key. Once you have improved the sensory pathways – your own co-ordination between the brain and vagina and then improved its strength with the Gyneflex™ - you need to be able to incorporate that into your lovemaking and that is where the challenge begins. I usually tell my clients that they should just tell their partner, tongue in cheek, "I'm working/concentrating!" You start by co-ordinating one position at a

14

time, mastering that one and then progressing onto the next. The position that is usually the easiest for women to get a good grip on their partner is on all fours, with your partner penetrating you from behind. You have the assistance of gravity and are able to use your breathing freely which is crucial for increased tension. Each time your partner re-enters the vaginal canal it is your opportunity to apply tension around the penis, increasing the sensation for you both. He may not last long if you get it right, but it will be an amazing and empowering experience for you.

Other Ways of Exercising Pelvic Floor Muscles

◆ Biofeedback. All clients that come through my clinic are measured with a biofeedback probe inserted into the vagina. This allows both the client and myself to see first-hand just what activity and strength exists within their vagina. It is a powerful tool that not only shows their progress weekly from thereon, but empowers them towards their goal. The biofeedback is a useful tool, which, when linked to a computer allows for a number of programs to be used for assessing, training and conditioning in both the contraction and relaxation phase.

◆ Electrical stimulation. Sometimes a special electrical device is used to stimulate the pelvic floor muscles with the aim of making them contract and become stronger. Whilst this may be needed in extreme cases, it is essential to teach the client how to activate the floor using their own sensory cells.

◆ Vaginal cones. These are small plastic cones that you put inside your vagina for about 15 minutes, twice a day. The cones come in a set of different weights. At first, the lightest cone is used. You need to use your pelvic floor muscles to hold the cone in place, thus helping you to exercise your pelvic floor muscles. Once you can hold onto the lightest one comfortably, you move up to the next weight, and so on.

Use *Pelvic Floor Secrets* as a reference, an exercise program and a lifestyle choice. Mature with a renewed confidence in your ability to remain in control, empowered, sexy and confident. For me, 50 is the new 40! I love that I am vain enough to want to remain sexy, able to wear the beautiful dresses I have in my wardrobe, not having to give them to someone else to look good as I buy a new wardrobe that does nothing for my confidence. My personal summers continue to drive me mad, but my sex life is alive, very much so, and I have that spring in my step that allows me to enjoy each day. I wish you the same success as you use the book to 'get back to sexy' and enjoy your life.

God bless x

14

Glossary

Abdominal	The muscles that form the wall of he abdomen; our midsection of the trunk.
Anatomical position	Referring to the original/correct position of \ the organs within the body.
Bladder	The organ (sac) inside the pelvic area used for storing urine.
Blackwall Tunnel	Four lane traffic underpass linking north and south London.
Bartholin's glands	Part of the greater vestibular gland the size of a pea just outside the opening of the vagina.
Clitoris	Organ of erectile tissue at the top of the vagina, which becomes swollen when correctly stimulated and can result in orgasm.
Continence	The ability to prevent involuntary urination and/or bowel movements; it is also the ability to control physical (especially sexual) implulses allowing for self-restraint, moderation or abstinence.

Diaphragm   A curved muscular membrance that separates the abdomen from the area around the lungs.

Fascia   Connective tissue surrounding muscle or groups of muscles, blood vessels and nerves, binding some structures together, while allowing others to slide smoothly over each other.

Incontinence   The inability to control involuntary urination or bowel movements; a lack of sexual restraint or self-control – literally a lack of moderation of an action or emotion.

Idiopathic   Relating to a disease having no known cause, or a disease that is not the result of any other disease.

Kinesiology   The study of mechanics of motion with respect to human anatomy. It allows for muscle testing that reveals and corrects musculoskeletal imbalances and identifies food sensitivities.

Levator   A muscle that helps to lift the body part to which it is attached.

Levator Ani   Two part muscle: front part also known as pubococcygeus – sling that pulls the rectum, vagina and urethra anteriorly towards the pubic bones. The second is known as the illiococcygeus – a horizontal sheet that assists in the support of the pelvic viscera.

Laxity

A slackening or looseness of a muscle(s), lack of tautness, firmness or rigidity within it. It can also relate to a displacement in the motion of a joint as in SPD.

Multifidus

Lying just under the erector spine, this muscle has many lobe shaped segments and is the true stabiliser of the lower back.

Neurological

The function of the nervous system affecting both nerve and muscle tissue.

Oblique

Slanting muscles in the midsection, which support the ribcage.

Pelvic Diaphragm

The portion of the floor of the pelvis formed by the coccygeal and levator ani muscles and their fasciae.

Prostatitis

Inflammation of the prostate gland.

Rectus

Abdominal Rectus being any straight muscle, is the upper part of the abdominal structure.

Stabilisation

The act or process of keeping something in place; maintaining balance.

Transverse Abdominal   Lower section of the abdominal lying and extending crosswire (left to right).

Umbilicus   Navel/belly button.

Urethra   The short tube above the vagina that connects the bladder to the outer side of the body.

Vajazzle   To give the female external genitals a sparkly makeover with crystals in order to enhance the appearance.

Vajayjay   Urban 21st century name for vagina.

Vestibular bulbs   The erectile tissue that becomes swollen during sexual arousal.

Viscera   The internal organs in the body, especially those of the abdomen such as the intestines.

Visceroptosis   Prolapse or a sinking of the abdominal viscera away from their natural (anatomical) position.

References and further reading:
Chek P, How to Eat, Move and be Healthy
Waterhouse D, Outsmarting the Female Fat Cell
Woolcott W, The Metabolic Typing Diet

Recipe

Ghee (Clarified Butter)

Ghee is often used in Indian cooking – it adds a delicious rich flavour to recipes. Ghee has a much higher smoking point than butter, so is very useful for frying. It also keeps longer than butter.

250g unsalted butter, diced roughly 1.5 cm size

1. Make your own butter (see page 29 of "Fast and Easy Indian Cooking") or use bought unsalted butter. Using the built-in electronic weighing scales, weigh the butter into the Thermomix bowl. Cook 7 to 10 minutes/60°C/Speed 1. The butter should boil and become a clear golden liquid. (If you're using the ghee for Indian cooking rather than pelvic lubricating, add a curry leaf in the last minute of cooking if desired.)

2. Leave to cool, then pour the golden liquid carefully through a very fine sieve into a sterilized jar and throw away the white milk solids that were left behind. Cover with a sterilized lid and keep in the fridge.

Quick Reference Index

Continence Foundation:
www.continence-foundation.org.uk
email: info@continence-
foundation.org.uk

Bladder and Bowel Foundation:
Bladder & Bowel Foundation
SATRA Innovation Park
Rockingham Road
Kettering, Northants, NN16 9JH
Helpline: 0845 345 0165
General enquiries: 01536 533255
Fax: 01536 533240
Email: info@
bladderandbowelfoundation.org

Hard Flaccid:
www.hardflaccid.org

**Chartered Institute of
Physiotherapy:**
14 Bedford Row
London WC1R 4ED
Tel: 020 7306 6666 (or +4420 7306
6666 from outside the uK).
www.csp.org.uk

Association of Prostate Awareness:
Newham African Caribbean
Resource Centre
627/633 Barking Road
Plaistow
London E13 9EZ
Tel: 0208 471 2258
Email: sonia.harding@prostate-
awareness.co.uk

Center for Vaginal Health:
New York Downtown Hospital
Wellness and Prevention Centre
170 William Street
New York, NY 10038
Phone: 646-588-2500
Fax: 646-588-2689
Email: info@
centerforvaginalhealth.com

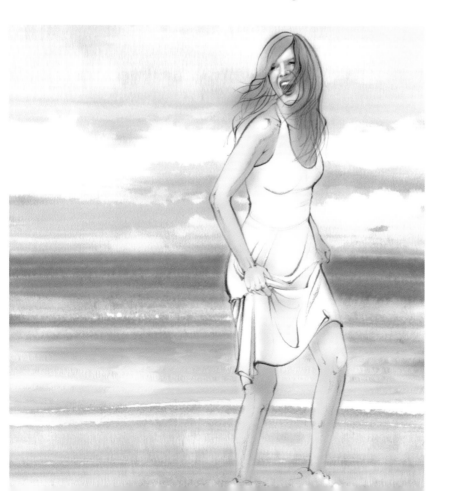